MW01070461

DIET-STEP®

20 GRAMS/20 MINUTES

FOR WOMEN ONLY!

OTHER BOOKS BY THE AUTHOR:

WALK, DON'T RUN. Philadelphia: Medical Manor Press, 1979.

THE DOCTOR'S WALKING BOOK. New York: Ballantine Books, 1980.

THE DOCTOR'S WALKING DIET. Philadelphia: Medical Manor Books®, 1982.

DIETWALK®: THE DOCTOR'S FAST 3-DAY SUPERDIET. Philadelphia: Medical Manor Books®, 1983. Pocket Books® edition, Simon & Schuster, New York, 1987.

WALK, DON'T DIE. Philadelphia: Medical Manor Books®, 1986. Bart Books edition: New York, 1988.

WALK TO WIN: THE EASY 4-DAY DIET & FITNESS PLAN. Philadelphia: Medical Manor Books®, 1990.

Medical Manor Books® are available at special quantity discounts for sales promotions, premiums, fund raising or educational use. Book excerpts can also be created to fit special needs.

For details write the Special Markets Dept. of Medical Manor Books®, 3501 Newberry Road, Philadelphia, PA 19154.
    Phone: 800-DIETING (343-8464)
    Fax: 215-440-WALK (9255)
    E-mail: medicalmanor@aol.com
    Website: www.diet-step.com or www.medicalmanorbooks.com

DIET-STEP®

20 GRAMS/20 MINUTES

FOR WOMEN ONLY!

BY

Fred A. Stutman, M. D.

MEDICAL MANOR BOOKS®

Philadelphia, PA

DIET-STEP®
20 GRAMS/20 MINUTES - FOR WOMEN ONLY!

Copyright© 2001 by Fred A. Stutman, M.D.

All Rights Reserved. No part of this book may be reproduced, copied or utilized in any form or by any means, electronic, mechanical, photocopying, recording, or by any information storage and retrieval system, without permission in writing from the publisher. Inquiries should be addressed to: Medical Manor Books®, 3501 Newberry Road, Philadelphia, PA 19154.

MEDICAL MANOR BOOK® is the registered trademark of Manor House Publications, Inc. **REG. U.S. PAT. OFF.**

DR. WALK® is the registered trademark of Dr. Stutman's Diet & Fitness Newsletter. **REG. U.S. PAT. OFF.**

DIET-STEP® is the registered trademark of Dr. Stutman's 20 Grams/20 Minutes Weight-Loss and Fitness Program. **REG. U.S. PAT. OFF.**

FIT-STEP® is the registered trademark of Dr. Stutman's Fitness Walking Program. **REG. U.S. PAT. OFF.**

TRIM-STEP® is the registered trademark of Dr. Stutman's Stretching and Strength Training Program. **REG. U.S. PAT. OFF.**

Library of Congress Cataloging-in-Publication Data

Stutman, Fred A.
  Diet-Step : 20 grams/20 minutes : for women only / by Fred A. Stutman. --
    1 st ed. p. cm.
  Includes index.
  ISBN 0-934232-10-5 (Cloth) -- ISBN 0-934232-09-1 (Paper)
  1. Women--Health and hygiene. 2. Physical fitness for women. 3. Reducing diets. 4. Women--Nutrition. I Title.

RA778.S9245 2000
613.7'045--dc21   00-034857

First Edition 2001
Manufactured in the United States of America

To:

Suzanne

Robert, Mary, Samantha, Alana

Roni, Geoffrey

Craig, Christine

&

Sparky

AUTHOR'S CAUTION

IT IS ESSENTIAL THAT YOU CONSULT YOUR OWN PHYSICIAN BEFORE BEGINNING THIS DIET AND EXERCISE PROGRAM.

Fred A. Stutman, M.D.

ACKNOWLEDGEMENTS

EDITOR: Dr. Suzanne Stutman

MANAGING EDITOR: Patricia McGarvey

EDITORIAL STAFF: Mary Ann Johnston, Linda Quinn, Sheryl Bartkus, Patti Hartigan, Kathy Bradley, Regina Varano, Ellen V. Henry

PERMISSIONS: Greta Blackburn, Editor, Ms. Fitness Magazine; Andrée Broudo, President, Atlas Multimedia Corp.; J & J Snack Foods, Inc (Superpretzel®); Alexander Leaf, M.D. Professor Emeritus, Clinical Medicine, Harvard Medical School; Phyllis Deutsch, Editor, University Press of New England; Carol A. Verdi, M.D.; Medical Times - Romaine Pierson Publishers, Inc.; Physician's Health Bulletin; Sorosh Roshan, M.D., M.P.H., President of the National Council of Women/U.S.A., and President of the International Health Awarness Network

CARTOONS: Reg Hider, Norm Rockwell.

WORD PROCESSING: Accu-Med Transcription Service (Shelly Green and Paul Fowler), Southampton, PA.

TYPOGRAPHY + GRAPHIC DESIGN: Alexander E. Shin, Sir Speedy Graphic Design, Philadelphia, PA.

COVER DESIGN: Geralynne Slowe

BOOK PRODUCTION: RR Donnelley & Sons Co.

PUBLISHER: Medical Manor Books®, Philadelphia, PA.

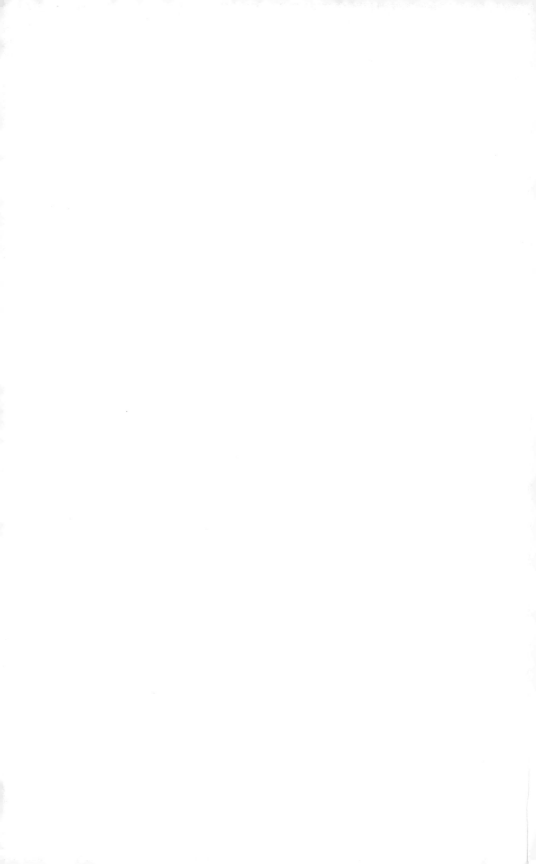

TABLE OF CONTENTS

INTRODUCTION

The problem with most diet and exercise programs is that they are too complicated and too time consuming. Most of these plans do not take into consideration that everyone has a life to lead that is packed full of hundreds of things to do each week. Women in particular, with their busy schedules, do not really have the time to follow time-consuming diet and fitness programs.

Diet-Step: 20 Grams/20 Minutes is the first medically formulated diet and fitness plan for women of all ages, all body builds and all levels of physical fitness. I have developed this program exclusively for my female patients, for my wife and her friend Phyllis, who you will meet in Chapter 1, and for my daughter, who like most of you wants a diet and fitness plan that is easy to follow, safe and effective and does not interfere with day to day living. In the Diet-Step® plan for women only, there are no calories or grams of carbohydrates to count, no diet clinics to report to, no difficult meals to prepare, no prepackaged dehydrated foods to buy and no yucky protein drinks to gag on. There are no expensive fitness clubs to join, no special equipment or clothing to purchase, no trying to keep up with a 20 year old robotic fitness instructor and no strenuous back-breaking exercises to endure.

Diet-Step: 20 Grams/20 Minutes is a healthful, life-long diet and fitness plan for weight loss, weight control, good health, physical fitness and a trim, well sculptured body. This plan is easy to follow, safe and effective, and works quickly to help you lose weight, achieve maximum physical fitness and develop a shapelier figure. And what's more, it will keep you in excellent health and help you live longer, while you look and feel younger. Try it! You'll like it! It works!

DIET-STEP® is not just another diet program!
DIET-STEP® is not just another fitness plan!
DIET-STEP® is not just another pretty face!
****
DIET-STEP® is for women only!

STEP 1:
DIET-STEP®

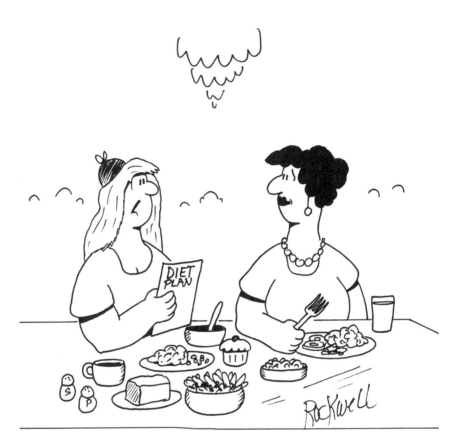

**"LOW CARBOHYDRATE, HIGH PROTEIN,
LOW FAT -- I'M CONFUSED!"**

CHAPTER 1

20 GRAMS/20 MINUTES: FOR WOMEN ONLY!

****

PHYLLIS AND SUE'S DIET ADVENTURE

As I sat across the dinner table from my wife Sue (a college pro-fessor) and her friend Phyllis (a prominent book editor), I was both amazed and mystified by their dinner conversation. Both of them have currently been on separate diet programs for the past three months. Sue is on one of the many low-carbohydrate diets, where she counts each and every gram of carbohydrate that she consumes. Phyllis, on the other hand, is on one of the popular diet programs where they count calories with each and every meal. Both Sue and Phyllis have probably lost and regained over 10 pounds over the past several months, but each is determined to stick to her respec-tive diet plans, no matter what the consequences. Their dinner con-versation went something like this:

Sue: "I really don't think I've lost that much weight on this low carbohydrate diet over the past few months."

Phyllis: "You really look a lot thinner to me, Sue."

Sue: "Do I really, Phyllis? Well, maybe I did lose some weight because my jeans are loose in the waist. You look a lot thinner since the last time I saw you a few months ago."

Phyllis: "I have lost some weight, but this counting calories with every meal is starting to get on my nerves, and there are times when I wish I could have a nice, juicy hamburger."

Sue:	"That's the great part of my diet Phyllis. I can eat all of the meat that I want."
Phyllis:	"You really can eat any quantity of meat?"
Sue:	"Yes. In fact, I have bacon and eggs for breakfast, a hamburger for lunch, of course without the roll, and a juicy steak for dinner. However, I can't have bread, potatoes or vegetables with the steak. It's actually pretty boring."
Phyllis:	"Well, my diet lets me have most of the vegetables that I want, and bread if I want it, but unfortunately, I can't have a steak, because I'll exceed the number of calories that I'm allowed to have. You know, I really miss the meat."
Sue:	"And I really miss the bread and vegetables, not to mention the fruit that I'm not allowed to have."
Phyllis:	"That's the good part of my diet. I can have a certain number of fruits and vegetables per day, just as long as they don't go over the allotted number of calories."
Sue:	"Well, aside from that, what would you like to order, Phyllis?"
Phyllis:	"Well, how about the lobster with ginger sauce?"
Sue:	"That sounds great, Phyllis. And let's order the steamed greens and sautéed string beans with garlic."
Phyllis:	"Sounds delicious. How about adding the shrimp and asparagus in garlic sauce?"
Sue:	"Wonderful! I don't think I'll have any soup, then."
Phyllis:	"How about splitting an order of dumplings?"
Sue:	"Great! And I think I'll have a Chinese beer."
Phyllis:	"Me, too. That sounds great."
Sue:	"I wonder how many carbs the dumplings have?"
Phyllis:	"I wonder how many calories are in the dumplings?"
Sue:	"I guess it doesn't matter that much, since the lobster and shrimp are both steamed."
Phyllis:	"Yes, but they are probably fried in peanut oil, and that's high in fat."

Sue: "There's probably sugar in the sauce, and that would push my carb level way over the top."

Phyllis: "The amount of fat in the dumplings and sauces will certainly exceed my number of calories for today."

Sue: "But, aren't these dumplings yummy?"

Phyllis: "Very delicious

Sue: "Do you think you'll be back in town again soon?"

Phyllis: "Why, yes. I have a meeting in New York in two months, so we can meet for dinner again."

Sue: "This lobster is out of this world!"

Phyllis: "I can't get anything this good at any of the restaurants in New Hampshire. And the shrimp and asparagus are certainly delicious, too."

Sue: "I bet these string beans with garlic are full of hidden carbs, but aren't they wonderful?"

Phyllis: "They certainly are good, and I'm sure the vegetable content will offset any of the fat in the sauce."

Sue: "I know I'll never be able to get into my jeans tomorrow."

Phyllis: "It's important to drink at least eight glasses of water every day if you really want these diets to work."

Sue: "I don't think they mentioned drinking a lot of water in the book on this low carbohydrate diet."

Phyllis: "You better. I heard that a low carbohydrate diet can cause kidney damage, so you better drink at least six to eight glasses of water every day."

Sue: "I better get my cholesterol count checked, too. Since the diet is so high in fat, it worries me."

Phyllis: "That's the beauty of my diet. The calorie and fat content is low. Actually too low, when you come to think of it. Nothing much tastes any good without a little meat in it, or a little butter on the bread."

Sue: "I can have all the cheese and nuts I want on this diet, especially for snacks."

Phyllis: "That's pretty high in fat, Sue. My diet limits cheese and nuts to a bare minimum. You know, I really miss cheese, too."

Sue: "What I really miss are the fruits. That's the hardest part of this diet."

Phyllis: "And how about the vegetables?"

Sue: "You're right; I really miss them, too. I can only have a limited amount of vegetables on this diet."

Phyllis: "Unfortunately, I have to get weighed in every week and then get a lecture if I don't lose enough weight. I feel as if I'm back in school again."

Sue: "It sounds more like you're reporting to your parole officer or the weight-control police."

Phyllis: "You know that since my time is limited, I was thinking about changing to one of those diet plans where you buy all of their foods in advance."

Sue: "One of my friends is on a diet plan like that and she said that not only is it expensive, but that the food tastes like cardboard."

Phyllis: "This meal is fantastic! A gourmet's delight. I could eat like this every night."

Sue: "So could I."

Phyllis: "One thing we know for sure is that we can't have any dessert."

Sue: "Yes, I can't have the sugar carbs in desserts."

Phyllis: "And I can't have the calories in desserts."

Sue: "Phyllis, this meal was wonderful!"

Phyllis: "It really was special, even if we both went off our diets."

Sue: "I can't eat another thing!"

Phyllis: "Neither can I."

Sue: "I won't eat anything until breakfast."

Phyllis: "Neither will I."

Sue: "What would you like for breakfast, Phyllis?"

Phyllis: "Just some cereal and fruit."

Sue: (sighing) "All I can have is a cheese omelet with bacon."

Phyllis: "Yummy!"

SAY GOODBYE TO DIETING

Most women realize the ideal weight touted in women's magazines and in clothing advertisements is completely, 100% unobtainable. So often does the idea of losing weight obsess your psyche, that chronic anxiety and frustration, instead of weight loss is the result.

One of the main problems with dieting is the fact that women who are on diets binge-eat far more often than non-dieters. Dieters do not eat according to whether they feel hungry, but actually eat out of the false notion that they are being good or bad. If in fact they eat a dessert that they feel "is bad for them," then frustration and anxiety sets in and they take new oaths to be better. In effect then, it is not the dieter but it is the diet to be blamed.

When you start limiting your food intake, neurochemicals in the brain respond as if the body were starving itself. The metabolic rate slows down so that the body does not burn food as quickly in order to survive starvation. This deprivation in effect produces food cravings, which is exactly the opposite effect that you are trying to achieve. The psychological and physiological effects of dieting can therefore be devastating. In our culture it is very easy to not like our bodies. The mirror becomes the enemy, and we feel captured in our reflections. It is only natural then that we feel if we deprive ourselves we will then be released from the prison in the mirror.

According to behavioral psychologists, children left to themselves will select a variety of foods and when they have had enough they stop eating. Adults, on the other hand, identify foods as either being good (healthy) or bad (unhealthy), and attempt, although usually not successfully, to make their selection from them. The road to normal eating is to stop listening to the myriad of advice about what to eat and start to follow your own biological and physiological needs for essential nutrients. We all know that fruits, vegetables, grains and fish are good for you; however, you must tune up your psychological motor to actually make pleasurable choices.

Snacking on occasion on junk food is inevitable, and as long as you do not beat yourself up over it, you will survive nicely. If on the other hand snacks are restricted permanently then your brain's neurochemicals and transmitters will send you into a binge-eating frenzy. Once satisfied with a small self-satisfying snack, your brain will leave you alone for a relatively long time.

Remember, you live in your body and you do not have to make drastic changes in order to feel good about yourself. The 20/20 Diet-Step® plan will enable you to lose as much weight as you want to in order to feel comfortable with your body. You will no longer be a prisoner in your mirror. Learn to love your body even before you go on the Diet-Step® program. There is no doubt that you will love it more when you have completed the program, but do not underestimate your current good looks, sex appeal and body contours. All women, by nature, are beautiful and you should feel beautiful and self-confident inside. I have never met a woman who is not beautiful.

Before we start the Diet-Step® 20 grams/20 minutes program for women only, here are a few preliminary steps to make your diet and exercise program more enjoyable:

1. Step into the Diet-Step® plan which lets you lose weight at your own pace without complicated diet plans, counting calories, fad diets or starvation techniques. The plan is relatively easy and quite effective in losing weight quickly and maintaining weight loss. The Diet-Step® 20/20 Plan is as crystal clear as 20/20 eyesight.

2. Take that next step in the Fit-Step® plan for energy, fitness and pep. The Fit-Step® plan of only 20 minutes of aerobic exercise (walking) six days per week will keep a fresh supply of oxygen surging through your blood vessels to all of your body's hungry cells. You will look and feel better and actually be healthier and live longer on the Fit-Step® plan.

3. Next, step into the Trim-Step® plan, which includes strength resistance exercises, 20 minutes two days a week. This plan, in addition to helping you lose weight and feel and look better, will actually sculpt and mold all of your body's muscles and give you a perfect figure. There is no need to do strenuous exercises or power weight lifting in order to get the perfect body for you. This plan is designed with you in mind and ease of use. Try it, you'll like it.

4. And lastly, take "beauty steps" to accentuate your feelings of happiness and well-being. Buy a new dress, a sweater or a new pair of shoes. Get a flattering haircut and make-up in colors that compliment your complexion. Get some flowers for your desk at work or for a table at home. Smile, it feels good! Smiling makes you feel and look great, and helps to keep anxiety and depression at bay. Listen to music whenever possible, and sing along whether your voice is good or bad. Now you are probably saying, what does all of this have to do with dieting and exercise? Absolutely nothing in theory, but everything in practice. When you feel good about yourself, you will feel great about the way that you look and feel and that has everything to do with the Diet-Step® weight loss and fitness plan. Fun, flowers, smiling, music and feeling good - what could be wrong with that!

FOOD, FUEL AND ENERGY

I.   HOW YOUR BODY BURNS CALORIES (FUEL)

A. BASAL METABOLIC RATE: Just eating food burns calories! Sounds too good to be true, but it actually is a fact.
Your body burns up calories from the food that you eat
(carbohydrate, fat and protein) and turns part of it into fuel
that you need to function every day. Protein, carbohydrate
and fat each burn a different amount of calories in this conversion process. If your body realizes there are not enough
calories in your diet, it switches on to a slower metabolic
rate in an attempt to protect you from starvation, as in times
of famine -- it's a natural physiologic reaction.

Unfortunately, obese people stay in the slow metabolic rate mode because they usually go on and off diets
frequently, wherein the body's weight rebounds very gradually. The metabolic rate, therefore, stays in the slow mode,
because the body never knows when it will get enough food
to sustain life. Then, at times when there are excess calories
in your diet, weight is easily gained because your metabolism is stuck in the slow mode.

B. EXERCISE: The most important way to burn calories is by
exercise. This certainly is a more efficient method of losing
weight than by just relying on your body to burn calories by
the sedentary process of just eating food. (Remember, just
the act of eating food with no exercise whatsoever, burns a
certain amount of calories.)

1. Fast, quick, physical exercise such as jogging, tennis,
basketball, aerobics and race walking burns primarily
carbohydrate stores in the production of energy.

2. Slow, repetitive physical activity such as walking and swimming burns primarily fat stored in the body, which is the best type of exercise for sustained weight loss.

C. FOODS THAT WE EAT: In general, we burn almost all of the protein and carbohydrates that we eat every day. We store the remaining carbohydrates in our muscles and liver in the form of a chemical compound called glycogen. This glycogen is used for the future production of energy. The difference between the energy supplied by protein and carbohydrate in our diets and our total energy needs each day has to come from burning fats.

Weight gain actually occurs from taking in more calories in the form of dietary fats than were burned off as fuel for energy. On a low-fat diet, calories are removed from storage in fat cells and are added to the fuel mixture of protein and carbohydrate for the production of energy. This results in steady, permanent weight loss, unlike the temporary water weight loss of low-carbohydrate, high-protein diets. It's simple -- less fat taken in results in more storage fat being burned as fuel, resulting in lovely, thin fat cells remaining! More fat taken in results in more fat being stored, and less fat being burned, and lumpy, unsightly fat cells remaining!

II.   HOW YOUR BODY CHANGES FOOD INTO ENERGY

A. PROTEIN in our diet is not a significant factor in weight regulation. Almost all of the energy contained in the protein that you eat is burned as fuel for the body's metabolic process of functioning (living). Hardly any of the calories contained in dietary protein is converted into fat storage. Only 75% of the energy contained in protein can be used for your metabolic processes such as repairing the body cells, because it takes almost 25% of the energy in protein just to change it into a form that our body can use to build and repair the body's cells, tissues and organs.

B. FAT, on the other hand, is easily converted into energy. Whereas almost none of the calories contained in protein in our diets is converted into fat cells (storage), almost 95% of the dietary fat calories can be stored in fat cells when you take in excess calories of fat in your diet. In other words-it is the fat in your diet that makes you fat! It is not necessarily the number of calories in your diet that makes you fat, it is the number of fat calories that makes you fat.

DANGEROUS DIETING

So, the very first question that comes to mind is, then how come people lose weight on all of those popular low-carbohydrate, high-fat diets? For example, they say you can have bacon and eggs for breakfast, hot dogs for lunch, and a juicy steak for dinner. Sounds tempting, doesn't it? They also tell you that you can't have any, or at the very least, limited amounts of carbohydrates with each meal. For instance - no vegetables, fruits, cereals, breads, potatoes, pasta, etc. Sounds unappetizing and unhealthy, doesn't it? It certainly is!

The simple fact is, that you do lose weight, initially, on these very low carbohydrate, high fat, high protein diets; however, most of the initial weight loss is water weight loss, due to a metabolic process called ketosis, which in fact is a condition found in unhealthy patients (for example: diabetes and kidney disease) not in healthy people. Once the body gets rid of the water, it starts burning fat, which is left over -- which, in itself, is a good thing; however, the downside is that this abnormal process of ketosis also begins to burn the body's protein (muscle tissue). This is a very bad thing. By attempting to burn protein as a source of fuel or energy, the body is actually breaking down the most important element in the body that is used to sustain life (building and repairing the body's tissues, cells and organs). The fact that a substance called ketones appears in your urine (a by-product of this abnormal process called ketosis), shows you clear evidence that your body is breaking down its muscle tissue. This is one of the reasons that fatigue and general weakness have been reported as early side effects of this completely unhealthy diet. Also, kidney and liver damage may result if too much of the body's protein is broken down in these unhealthy, high-protein, high-fat, low-carbohydrate diets.

And to make matters worse, these diets are deficient in vitamins, minerals and essential nutrients.

These rapid weight loss programs (low-carbohydrate, high-fat, high-protein diets) also have the added downside of what's called "rebound weight gain." This occurs after the initial weight loss, which results from fat and protein breakdown used for energy production (fuel). The body's carbohydrate stores then become depleted because of the very low intake of carbohydrates in these diets, and thus, there is limited availability of carbohydrate to be burned as a fuel. Unfortunately, these low stores of carbohydrates are designed to be the very first type of calories to be burned as fuel in our normal metabolism.

Once your body becomes aware that it is carbohydrate depleted by exhibiting the symptoms of fatigue, malaise, muscle cramps, and decreased urine output, which occurs after the initial water loss, then your brain's control center receives stress (SOS) signals from all of the body's cells suffering from carbohydrate depletion. What these cells are telling your brain is, "We need complex carbohydrates in order to function properly. We can no longer tolerate our cells' protein being burned as fuel. We need to preserve out protein for the proper metabolic function of our cells in order to live a healthy life. We are warning you (brain) that there is no compromise in these demands, for to be foolhardy and overlook basic physiology will be the death of us all, including all of you brain cells. Then who's going to do the thinking for the rest of us?"

Once your brain's central control center receives this flood of distress messages, it immediately calls a top-level brain cell emergency meeting. These CEO brain cells unanimously react with an overwhelming majority vote (100 billion to 1) that the body had better get a cheaper source of fuel (complex carbohydrate) or they face complete annihilation. The one dissenting vote, of course, was a damaged brain cell, which occurred from the lack of oxygen caused by this unhealthy diet. The message is then sent out loud and clear from your brain's satiety (hunger) center - and it says "Feed me - feed me carbohydrates!" Just when you're feeling exhausted and done in by this enemy diet, your hunger center sets you off on a <u>carbohydrate binge</u> - you just can't help it! And even though the brain's smartest cells are only telling the body's cells that all they need is a cheap, ready source of fuel for energy (complex carbohydrates), all they can actually hear, feel, smell and sense is "Now, I need cake, candy, pie, chocolate and sweets to counteract this lethargy I've been feeling for weeks or months." And then what happens is that your body explodes into its former fat self and then some, hence the term "REBOUND WEIGHT GAIN."

Eventually, your sweet tooth gets satisfied, and you resume your former unhealthy diet of excess fat and low carbohydrates. Not a pretty picture, is it? And yet, over 75% of the commercially available diet books work on this abnormal metabolic process principle. Well, enough said. Now let's talk about what constitutes a healthy diet and one that we can actually lose weight on, quickly and easily, without side effects.

C. <u>CARBOHYDRATES</u>: Before we can discuss a healthy weight loss program, we have to talk briefly about carbohydrates. Carbohydrate is the body's natural source of fuel to produce energy. One of the most important basic metabolic functions of the body is to use almost all of the carbohydrate calories you eat, as a source of fuel for energy production.

The left over carbohydrate calories not immediately used for fuel to produce energy are stored in your liver and your muscles as a product called "glycogen," which is stored as a ready source of fuel whenever the body needs it. It is readily available and can be retrieved from the liver and muscles into the blood stream easily, where it is quickly converted to a substance called glucose (sugar), where it then becomes available to burn as a fuel for energy production.

The best part of all is that only 5 to 10% of the carbohydrate that you eat is converted as storage into fat cells. That amounts to almost 90% being available for immediate or reserve fuel for energy production, without hardly any of the carbohydrate that you eat being converted into fat. To put it simply - complex carbohydrates in your diet will not make you fat!

Your body expends $2^{1}/_{2}$ times more energy converting dietary carbohydrate calories from your intestines into your blood stream for immediate energy use, and then into glycogen storage in your muscles and liver, than it takes to convert fat into a source of fuel for energy production. This means that almost all of the excess fat calories that you eat are stored in fat cells, and end up staying there indefinitely.

In other words, a high complex carbohydrate, low-fat diet causes your body to work harder after each meal burning calories for energy, than does a high-fat, low-carbohydrate diet. This means that your basal metabolic rate (the rate at which your body operates all of its functions) is considerably higher on the high-carbohydrate, low-fat diet. This higher basal metabolic rate results in an additional burning of approximately 250 calories daily by the simple thermic effect of converting carbohydrates into energy.

This higher basal metabolic rate can even be increased to an even faster rate with the addition of more complex carbohydrates in the diet. Of course, this cannot go on indefinitely, since it will eventually reach a saturation point by consuming too many carbohydrate calories. This then, would result in the glycogen storage sites in the liver and the muscle tissue becoming overfilled. Then the leftover carbohydrate calories would be converted to fat stores, which is certainly not desirable for weight reduction or weight maintenance.

III.   **HOW YOUR BODY STORES FUEL**

A. <u>FAT</u>: Fat is stored in fat cells (adipose tissue) in a ratio of four parts fat and one part water. Since there are <u>nine calories in each gram of fat,</u> it means that <u>one pound of fat contains 3500 calories!</u> It therefore takes a deficit of 3500 calories to lose just one pound of fat. Not a very pretty picture.

Fat, unfortunately, can be stored in unlimited quantities. Normal weight individuals have almost 100,000 calories stored in fat cells. By increasing fat in the diet, combined with a sedentary life style, it is quite easy to add another 50,000 to 100,000 calories in fat stores, increasing your weight 15 to 30 pounds every year. The only way to lose even one pound of body weight is to burn approximately 3500 calories. This can only be accomplished by cutting back on the amount of fat in the diet, and by increasing physical activity. Nothing else works! One of my favorite sayings to my patients when they ask me how to lose weight is: <u>"The only way you can lose weight is to eat less and walk more, or you can walk more and eat less!"</u>

B. <u>CARBOHYDRATE</u>: Carbohydrates that we eat are changed into a type of sugar (<u>glucose </u>in the bloodstream) to be used as an immediate source of fuel for the production of energy. Since only a small amount of the carbohydrates we eat is changed into immediate fuel sources, the majority of the carbohydrates consumed are changed into glycogen for storage in the liver and muscles. Remember, there are <u>only 4 calories in each gram of carbohydrate</u> (not nine calories as in fat).

Glycogen is stored in the liver and muscles in a ratio of <u>one part glycogen to four parts water</u> (just the opposite of fat storage which is four parts fat to one part water). The liver's capacity to store glycogen is limited to approximately 500 calories and the muscles can store about 1500 calories. Muscle tissue, however, can store extra calories when you exercise so that your muscles burn energy more efficiently. When you increase your glycogen stores by 500 calories, you will gain a pound of body weight and when you decrease your glycogen stores by 500 calories, you will lose a pound of body weight. This weight, as you can see from the above ratio of glycogen to water, is mostly water weight.

<u>Low carbohydrate diets</u>, as we have seen, cause glycogen depletion, and result in rapid water weight loss. When you decrease carbohydrates in your diet, you deplete your stores of glycogen rather quickly, since you only have 2000 calories stored as glycogen (500 in the liver and 1500 in the muscles), and therefore, the amount of water weight loss is limited. Once glycogen stores are low, then the body starts to burn fat slowly, which can take up to ten times as long as the water weight loss. Also, as previously stated, muscle tissue begins to be burned as fuel for energy on severely restricted carbohydrate diets. This results in a dangerous metabolic condition that we have discussed previously, known as ketosis. This is a condition that you don't

want to have. And once the body gets fed up with this abnormal diet, <u>rebound weight gain</u> occurs by leaps and bounds. As you'll see in the <u>Diet-Step® Plan</u>, you'll be eating a low fat diet with an abundance of high fiber complex carbohydrates, which will prevent ketosis and rebound weight gain from occurring.

DIET-STEP®: 20 GRAMS/20 MINUTES: FOR WOMEN ONLY!

The problem with most diet and exercise programs is that they are too complicated. There are too many tables to consult, to many diet meal plans to prepare and too many strenuous exercise programs with which to get comfortable. And above all, they are too time consuming. Most of these plans don't realize that everyone has a life to lead that is packed full of a hundred things to do each week. Women don't really have the time to follow any type of complicated or time-consuming diet or fitness program.

The beauty of the <u>Diet-Step® 20 Grams/20 Minutes Plan</u> is that it is designed especially for women who have limited amounts of time for diet and exercise, but who, on the other hand, would like a simple-easy-effective plan that doesn't interfere with the rest of their lives. Fortunately, Diet-Step 20 Grams/20 Minutes is just that plan. It's that simple! It's easy and it's effective. It doesn't take a lot of your valuable time, and it actually works!

I've developed this program exclusively for my female patients and also for my wife, her friend Phyllis, whom you have already met at the beginning of this chapter, and for my daughter, who, like most of you, wants a diet and exercise plan that doesn't interfere with day-to-day living. You'll be delighted at how easy the program is, and how well it works. My wife, who helped me edit most of my previous books, asked, "Can't you make this book easier to follow, sort of like a manual without all the rhetoric?"

Well, I guarantee that Diet-Step®: 20 grams/20 minutes will be easy to follow and will help you to lose weight, keep fit and trim and be healthy, too.

Women, as you and I both know, respond very differently to diet and exercise programs than men. Your metabolism is different, and your structural make-up is different, which requires a different type of exercise and diet plan made specifically for you. As many of you know, it is much harder for a woman to lose weight than it is for a man. The Diet-Step®: 20 Grams/20 Minutes Plan takes all of that into consideration in the formulation of your program.

Also, this diet and fitness program is geared towards a woman's body build, her metabolic rate, and her body composition. The exercise program has been designed for women's muscular strength, bone composition and ligament and tendon resiliency, which is entirely different from those of men. Women, although not physically as strong as men, pound for pound, have far greater endurance ability and this exercise program has been designed with that valuable asset in mind. A well-trained, physically fit, trim woman will be in far better shape for endurance activity than her male counterpart. Remember, this plan's for you. Give it six weeks, and I promise a thinner, fitter, trimmer you. All with a minimum of time and effort. The key to success here is consistency and adaptability -- two traits at which women excel.

DIET-STEP®: 20 Grams/20 Minutes is the first medically formulated diet and fitness program for women of all ages and body builds. No matter whether you're fat or thin, short or tall, athletic or unconditioned, young or old, muscular or flabby, coordinated or just a klutz -- this is the perfect diet and fitness plan for you.

Give me your tired, out of shape bodies, and I'll give you the new, improved you. There are no complicated diet plans to follow, no strenuous exercises to engage in, no special equipment to purchase and no health clubs or diet clinics to join. This is a truly simple, easy to follow, effective diet and fitness program with a minimum of time and effort on your part. Ok, enough rhetoric, let's get on with the program, so you can be thin, trim and fit quickly, and then get on with the rest of your lives.

DIET STEP®: 20 GRAMS/20 MINUTES - BASICS

The following is a summary of the DIET-STEP® 20 Grams/20 Minutes Plan, which is easy to follow and guaranteed to work. You can lose weight quickly or slowly depending on your own individual needs. You can maintain weight easily without the least bit of trouble. Actually the diet lets you have many of the fun foods and snacks that your body craves. There is no rebound weight gain and there are no inherent dangers to the diet plan itself, as opposed to the hazards inherent in low carbohydrate diets. You will lose weight quickly and easily.

DIET-STEP®: 20 GRAMS/20 MINUTES is a healthful, life-long diet and fitness plan for weight loss, weight control, good health, physical fitness and a trim, lean, sculptured body. As you will see in the following chapters, the plan is easy, inexpensive, safe, effective and works quickly to help you lose weight, achieve maximum physical fitness and develop a shapelier figure. And it will keep you in excellent health for the rest of your life.

DIET-STEP® is not just another diet program!
DIET-STEP® is not just another fitness plan!
DIET-STEP® is not just another pretty face!
* * * * * * *
DIET-STEP® is for women only!

Here are the **2 Basic Steps** of the **DIET-STEP®:**
20 GRAMS/20 MINUTE PLAN - FOR WOMEN ONLY!

STEP 1: DIET-STEP®

1. **20 Grams Fat/20 Grams Fiber daily - Quick Weight Loss Diet**
2. **No refined or processed foods - sugar, white flour, white rice**
3. **Limit salt, caffeine and alcohol**
4. **Drink at least six 8 oz. glasses of water daily**
5. **25-30 Grams Fat/25-30 Grams Fiber daily - Maintenance Weight Diet**

STEP 2: FIT-STEP®

1. **Walking 20 minutes daily, six days per week (or)**
2. **Indoor exercises (stationary bike, treadmill, etc.) 20 minutes daily, six days per week.**
3. **Walking 20 minutes daily, 5 days per week - Maintenance Fit-Step® Plan**
4. **Trim-Step® Walking Workout Exercises (strength training) 2 days per week.**

THAT'S ALL LADIES!

You'll see the details of the DIET-STEP® 20 Grams/20 Minutes Weight Loss & Fitness Plan unfold in the following chapters. It's really as easy as it sounds and what's more, it really works!

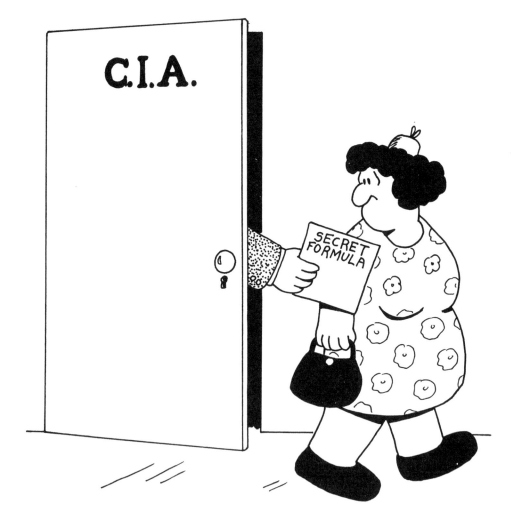

CHAPTER 2

QUICK WEIGHT LOSS: SECRET FORMULA!
****
20 GRAMS FAT/20 GRAMS FIBER

Diet-Step®: 20 Grams Fat/20 Grams Fiber is a quick and easy weight loss plan. No doubt about it! It is the only medically formulated diet plan for women that works and works and keeps on working. Weight loss is fast and easy, and what's more, it's permanent. There is no rebound weight gain: no food cravings, no starvation techniques, no liquid protein drinks and no diet pills. And no stuffing your face with meat, eggs, cheese, butter, cream, bacon, fat and more fat until you and your arteries are ready to explode.

The Diet-Step® Diet Plan is specifically designed for women of all ages, all shapes, all sizes and all weights. Diet-Step® is easy to follow and works quickly to shed all of the extra pounds that you want to lose. Here's all you have to do to lose weight for you.

QUICK WEIGHT LOSS
1. Eat 20 Grams Fat / 20 Grams Fiber daily
2. Do not eat refined or processed foods
   (sugar, white flour, white rice)
3. Limit salt, caffeine and alcohol
4. Drink at least six 8oz. glasses water daily
5. Walk 20 minutes, six days per week

WEIGHT-MAINTENANCE
1. Eat between 25-30 Grams Fat / 25-30-Grams Fiber daily
2. Walk 20 minutes, five days per week
3. Same #'s 2,3,4 above in quick weight loss plan.

THAT'S IT!

The **DIET-STEP® DIET PLAN** is a **high fiber diet** combined with a diet that is **low** in **total fat, saturated fat, cholesterol, salt** and **sugar.** When combined with a 20 minute daily walking program, it is the only diet that has been proven to be effective in weight loss, weight control, fitness and health maintenance.

The **high fiber** content of this diet provides a built-in mechanism against gaining weight and developing many diseases. At least 20 grams of fiber daily are required in the 20/20 Diet-Step® Plan. Eventually you can build up to 25-30 grams/day on the maintenance diet. See Fat & Fiber Counter in Chapter 6. By reducing the *total fat to 20 grams,* we eliminate many high fat calories that add extra weight and can block our arteries with saturated fat and cholesterol. The basis of this diet is **20 Grams Fat/20 Grams Fiber daily for quick weight loss.** The 20 grams of fat refers to total fat grams. These values can be found in the Fat & Fiber counter in Chapter 6.

Once you've reached your desired weight, then your weight can be maintained by switching to 25-30 grams fat/25-30 grams fiber. Then you'll be able to have all of those fun foods that you enjoy, like eggs, cheese, nuts, some oils, lean meats, pizza and a whole host of goodies and desserts without gaining an ounce. However, even while you're on the Quick Weight Loss diet you'll be able to have these tasty foods in moderation.

The *low refined sugar, flour, and rice* content of the diet eliminates simple, refined carbohydrates which have nutritionally deficient calories that add senseless pounds and may contribute to the development of heart disease and diabetes. Reducing the *salt content* also prevents excess accumulation of fluids and may help to prevent hypertension in susceptible people.

Even the amount of *caffeine* is limited in this diet since excess amounts of caffeine can stimulate the appetite center: the very thing we are trying to prevent. Excess caffeine can result in nervousness, insomnia, palpitations and headaches, and it may actually cause many breast, pancreas and heart disorders.

These factors are what makes the **DIET-STEP®** program effective in weight control, weight maintenance and disease prevention. Finally you have a diet that is as good for your insides as it is for your outsides. Here is a safe, effective diet and fitness program that can be continued for a lifetime, providing permanent weight control, good health and physical fitness. Remember, it's 20 grams total fat/20 grams of fiber for quick weight loss. For weight maintenance it's 25-30 grams fat/25-30 grams fiber. That's it! It's fast, easy and effective without counting calories or carbohydrate grams.

BASIC DIET-STEP® MEAL PLANS

The basic diet is divided into easy to follow meal plans. The diet meal plans have already factored in 20 grams total fat/20 grams fiber per day without having to add up grams of fat & fiber.

Once you've completed the first few weeks of your diet, the basic sample **DIET-STEP® MEAL PLANS** will become an automatic part of your everyday schedule. The diet is extremely easy to follow. There is no need to remember what to eat at home or what to order in a restaurant for any particular meal. Once you've become comfortable with the basic meal plans, you can then start to formulate your own individual meals by eating no more than 20 grams of total fat and no less than 20 grams of fiber daily. Consult the Fat and Fiber Counter in Chapter 6.

There is such a variety of foods included in this 20/20 diet that your taste buds will never tire of this healthful, nutritious, palatable diet program. By varying the foods in your diet, there are never any hunger pangs or food cravings. The Fat & Fiber Counter in Chapter 6 will allow you to mix and match any foods that you like. Remember, the **DIET-STEP® PLAN** is the only diet that in addition to controlling weight, will add years to your life by providing essential, healthful nutrients, antioxidants, phyto-nutrients, vitamins and minerals which eliminate harmful free-radical components from your body. This is a diet and exercise plan for fitness and health as well as for weight loss and weight control.

After you have reached your ideal weight on this easy diet program, you will never again have to worry about rebound weight gain. The **20/20 DIET-STEP®** plan enables you to lose weight quickly utilizing only these basic sample menu plans during your initial weight-loss program, or any combination of 20 grams of fat and 20 grams of fiber found in the <u>Fat and Fiber Counter.</u> You can lose weight quickly and safely with the basic **DIET-STEP® MEAL PLANS**. Just follow the easy meal plans and you will be trim and full of pep, when you do the **DIET-STEP®**. Remember, the <u>Quick-weight-loss Diet-Step® Plan is based on 20 grams total fat/20 grams fiber.</u>

MONDAY

BREAKFAST:
1   whole medium orange or 4 oz. (½ cup) fresh orange juice
1   slice whole wheat bread or whole wheat english muffin (½ teaspoon non-fat whipped/diet margarine without trans-fats or 1 tsp. jelly)
1-2   cups coffee or tea (artificial sweetener & non-fat milk)

LUNCH:
1   cup soup (vegetable, tomato, lentil, bean, pea, celery, minestrone, consommé, chicken noodle/rice, Manhattan clam chowder - no creamed or pureed soups) and 2-3 whole-wheat crackers.

1   tossed salad with lettuce, tomato and cucumber (lemon and/or 1 tsp. olive oil and vinegar or 1 tsp. non-fat dressing)
1   cup decaffeinated sugar free(coffee, tea or diet soda)
8   oz. glass water

MID - DAY SNACK:
1   Medium apple
8   oz. glass water

DINNER:
1   (4 oz.) tomato juice
1   LT/4C salad (lettuce, tomato, celery, carrot, cucumber, cauliflower), with non-fat dressing
3   oz. whole-wheat pasta primavera (fresh veggies and ½ cup marinara sauce)
1   slice whole-wheat bread/roll
4   oz. tomato or vegetable juice
8   oz. glass water

EVENING SNACK:
2   cups unbuttered, unsalted popcorn (hot air popcorn popper without oil)
8   oz. glass water

or

1   cup mixed fruits (berries, purple grapes, bananas)
8   oz. glass water

Total grams of fat: 19.1 Total grams of fiber: 25.8
WALK 20 MINUTES DAILY

TUESDAY

BREAKFAST:

½ medium grapefruit or 4 oz. (½ cup) fresh or unsweetened grapefruit juice

¾ cup cooked or cold whole grain (bran type) unsweetened cereal with ½ cup non-fat milk, 1/2 medium banana or 2 dozen raisins (½ oz.)

1-2 cup coffee or tea (artificial sweetener and non-fat milk)

LUNCH:

3 oz. (½ cup) tuna or chicken salad stuffed in whole- wheat pita bread (1 tsp. fat-free mayonnaise), with lettuce, toma-to and cucumber. Use tuna packed in water.

1 cup decaffeinated sugar-free (coffee, tea or diet soda)

8 oz. glass water

MID - DAY SNACK:

1 medium peach

8 oz. glass water

DINNER:

1 LT/4C salad with non-fat dressing (lettuce, tomato, celery, carrot, cucumber, cauliflower)

3 oz. baked or broiled fish (flounder, salmon, haddock, halibut, cod, sole, bass, bluefish, perch, trout) with lemon

1 medium baked potato or baked yam including skin (no butter, margarine or sour cream)

1 cup steamed vegetables (your choice)

4 oz. wine or 12 oz. light beer

8 oz. glass water

EVENING SNACK:

2   small unsalted, whole wheat pretzels, or one medium soft pretzel (Superpretzel®) with or without mustard

1   8 oz. glass lemonade (unsweetened)

or

¾   cup non-fat yogurt or low-fat fruit cottage cheese with 2 tsp. wheat germ or Miller's bran

8   oz. glass water

Total grams of fat: 18.0 Total grams of fiber: 20.0

WALK 20 MINUTES DAILY

- -

WEDNESDAY

BREAKFAST:

4   medium dried or stewed prunes or ½ cantaloupe or honeydew melon or 1 cup any fresh fruit

1   slice whole or cracked wheat bread (½ teaspoon whipped/diet oil-free margarine or 1 tsp. jelly)

1-2 cups coffee or tea (artificial sweetener and non-fat milk)

LUNCH:

1   cup fresh fruit salad on bed of lettuce with ½ cup low fat cottage cheese and 2 whole-wheat crackers

or

1   small chef salad with turkey (2 slices) and low-fat cheese (1 slice) only; use lemon, vinegar or 1 tsp. non-fat dressing

1   cup decaffeinated sugar free (coffee, tea or diet soda)

8   oz. glass water

MID - DAY SNACK:

1   medium pear

8   oz. glass water

DINNER:

1   LT/4C salad (lettuce, tomato, celery, carrot, cucumber, cauliflower), with non-fat dressing

3   oz. broiled or baked chicken breast, skin removed, add seasoning (paprika, garlic, pepper, etc.)

½   cup brown long whole grain rice; or ½ cup frozen corn or (1) small ear whole kernel corn (no butter, margarine, or salt)

1   cup steamed veggies (broccoli or spinach)

4   oz. tomato or vegetable juice

8   oz. glass water

EVENING SNACK:

1/8   slice angel food cake with non-fat whipped cream and sliced fruit or berries

1   8 oz. glass decaffeinated tea or soda (sugar free)

or

1   medium piece fresh fruit (apple, pear, peach, plum, banana, apricot or nectarine); or ½ cantaloupe or melon with ½ cup raspberries, strawberries or blueberries

8   oz. glass water

Total grams fat: 18.4 Total grams fiber: 22.3
WALK 20 MINUTES DAILY

THURSDAY

BREAKFAST:

1   whole medium orange or ½ cup fresh orange juice

¾   cup cold whole grain or bran cereal with ½ cup any fresh fruit & ½ cup non-fat milk

1-2 cups coffee or tea (non-fat milk and artificial sweetener)

LUNCH:

1   cup soup (any type except cream based) - the more vegetables and beans -the better.

1   whole wheat or multi-grain veggie sandwich with lettuce, tomatoes, sprouts, cucumber, carrots or any leafy green vegetable. Add Dijon mustard and sliced pickles.

1   glass decaffeinated sugar-free (coffee, tea, or soda)

8   oz. glass water

MID - DAY SNACK:

1   medium orange or tangerine

8   oz. glass water

DINNER:

Vegetable platter (broccoli, asparagus, squash, cauliflower, baked beans, carrots, green beans, spinach, mushrooms, stewed tomatoes) - choose any 4 (½ cup each)

1   whole-wheat dinner roll

4   oz. wine or 12 oz. light beer

8   oz. glass water

EVENING SNACK:

½   cup raisins with 2 tblsp. unsalted nuts

or

1   cup mixed fresh fruit (strawberries, blueberries, blackberries purple grapes, bananas, etc.)

8   oz. glass water

Total grams fat: 20.8 Total grams fiber: 21.0
WALK 20 MINUTES DAILY

- -

FRIDAY

BREAKFAST:
¾ cup cooked whole grain (oatmeal) or bran cereal with raisins (1/4 cup) or any fresh fruit, cinnamon, ½ cup non-fat milk
1 medium orange or ½ cup orange juice
1-2 cups coffee or tea (non-fat milk, artificial sweetener)

LUNCH:
1 slice pizza (tomato only or light cheese), topped with your choice of green peppers, mushrooms, onions, garlic, etc.
1 large tossed salad with non-fat dressing
12 oz. diet drink of your choice (decaffeinated and sugar-free)
8 oz. glass water

MID-DAY SNACK:
1 medium apple
8 oz. glass water

DINNER:
3 oz. baked eggplant or zucchini casserole parmesan baked with 1 tsp. olive oil and lightly breaded with whole wheat breading or 2 crumbled whole wheat crackers
1 cup steamed veggies (cauliflower, broccoli, spinach, etc.)
1 slice whole wheat bread or roll
4 oz. tomato or vegetable juice
8 oz. glass of water

EVENING SNACK:
½ cantaloupe or melon with ½ cup blueberries, strawberries or raspberries

8   oz. glass water

or

1   piece of fresh fruit (banana, pear, apple, peach, plum, orange or nectarine)

Total grams fat: 20.5 Total grams fiber: 22.0
WALK 20 MINUTES DAILY

- -

SATURDAY

BREAKFAST:
2   small whole grain pancakes (example: buckwheat - made with egg substitute) topped with fresh fruit or sugar-free syrup
½   cup (4 oz.) orange juice or 1 medium orange
1-2 cups coffee or tea (non-fat milk, artificial sweetener)

LUNCH:
Nicoise salad: tuna (dry), tomato, ½ sliced hard boiled egg, (3) black olives, (1) anchovy, onion, bell pepper, radish and celery (balsamic vinaigrette dressing on the side- just a few fork-fulls)
Diet drink of your choice (decaffeinated and sugar-free)
8   oz. glass water

MID-DAY SNACK:
1   small box raisins or ½ cup grapes (purple or green)
8   oz. glass water

DINNER:
3   oz. sirloin steak (lean) with grilled onions, mushrooms, garlic, peppers -your choice
1   medium baked potato or sweet potato with skin (no butter or sour cream)
1   cup steamed vegetables - your choice

4   oz. red wine or 12 oz. light beer

8   oz. glass water

EVENING SNACK:
¾ cup sugar-free, fat-free ice cream

or

Sugar-free jello with non-fat whipped cream

8   oz. glass water

Total grams fat: 20.1 Total grams fiber: 20.0
WALK 20 MINUTES DAILY

- -

SUNDAY

BREAKFAST:
2   eggs, (egg white or artificial egg omelet) with tomato, green peppers, onions and any non-fat cheese; or 1 poached or fried egg (non-fat, oil-free margarine - soft type)

½ cup orange or grapefruit juice

1   slice whole wheat, rye or pumpernickel bread with all fruit jam (1 tblsp.)

1- 2 cups coffee (non-fat milk, artificial sweetener)

LUNCH:
1   cup soup any type except creamed - the more veggies and beans the better

Large tossed salad with ½ tsp. oil & vinegar or non-fat dressing

2   whole-wheat crackers

Diet drink of your choice (decaffeinated and sugar-free)

8   oz. glass water

MID-DAY SNACK:
Any fruit

8   oz. glass water

DINNER:

3 oz. veal (lean) scaloppini or chicken (white meat without skin) cacciatore (baked with tomatoes, onions, peppers, mushrooms and garlic - your choice)

1 small baked or sweet potato with skin (no butter or sour cream)

1 slice whole wheat bread or roll

4 oz. tomato or vegetable juice

8 oz. glass water

EVENING SNACK:

1 cup mixed fruit (berries, bananas, peach, grapes, kiwi, etc.)

8 oz. glass water

or

1 baked apple (artificial sweetener) and cinnamon and raisins

Total grams fat: 20.7 Total grams fiber: 21.7

- - - - - - - - - - - - - REST! - - - - - - - - - - - -

DIET-STEP® NOTES

1. The above diets have all been pre-calculated to contain <u>no more than 20 grams of total fat and no less than 20 grams of fiber.</u> To formulate your own combination of foods, just check the values in the <u>Fat & Fiber counter</u> (Chapter 6) and mix and match any foods for any meals that you like. Remember to use no more than 20 grams of total fat and no less than 20 grams of fiber each day.

2. The most important part of the <u>Quick Weight-Loss Diet Plan</u> is to keep the total fat content to no more than 20 grams daily. Not only does this accelerate your weight loss, but you eliminate every known factor which can raise your blood cholesterol. By limiting your total fat to 20 grams daily, you in effect limit your intake of saturated fats, dietary cholesterol and trans-fatty acids - all of which

can significantly raise your blood cholesterol to dangerous levels. According to *The American Heart Association, for every 1% drop in blood cholesterol, your risk of a heart attack drops 2%.* Pretty impressive!

3. Another important factor in the 20 Grams Fat/20 Grams Fiber diet is that since the diet is primarily plant based, you will be eating lots of soluble and insoluble fiber (at least 20 grams), which are cholesterol fighters. These high fiber plants also contain numerous beneficial compounds including phyto-nutrients, antioxidants, flavinoids, B & C vitamins, minerals, beta and other carotenoids and folic acid, among others. All of these compounds help to fight heart disease, cancer and many other degenerative diseases.

4. You will notice that it is not necessary to count and record the grams of cholesterol with each meal. They are listed in the Fat & Fiber Counter for your own information. The American Heart Association usually recommends no more than 300 mg. per day. However, by limiting your total fat intake to 20 grams/day, you will be automatically limiting your total intake of cholesterol. There are a few exceptions that we'll discuss later; for example, shell fish, which is high in cholesterol, is not high in total grams of fat. Other fatty fishes like salmon, tuna, mackerel, herring, sardines and pompano, contain high amounts of 3-omega fatty acids which can significantly reduce your risk of heart disease. These 3-omega fatty acids are known as the heart-protecting fats.

5. Another exception to the high fat intake as a direct cause of heart disease is the fat content of seeds, nuts and certain oils (ex. olive oil). While these foods have a high total fat content, they are very low in saturated fats. They are also

high in mono-saturated fats, which also have been proven to be heart-protective. These foods can actually help to lower blood cholesterol and thereby reduce your risk of heart attacks. Nuts and seeds also contain many important vitamins and minerals, for example, selenium, which has been proven to be a potent cancer fighter. However, even these good fats have to be limited to some extent on the quick weight loss diet, since you can't exceed 20 grams of fat daily. You will, however, be able to add more of these fats on the maintenance diet.

6. You will also notice a column in the Fat & Fiber Counter (Chapter 6) marked saturated fats. These are the dietary fats that come from animal sources. These saturated fats are dangerous and can block the arteries in your heart, brain and legs. This blockage can lead to heart attacks, strokes and vascular disease. The American Heart Association recommends limiting saturated fats in women to 7-17 grams daily. However, it is not necessary to count the grams of saturated fat on the Diet-Step® Plan. By limiting the total grams of fat to 20 grams daily, your intake of saturated fats will be far below the recommended values. *Limit meat (beef, pork, veal) intake to no more than (2) small servings per week.*

7. After you've lost all of the weight that you wanted to lose on the Diet-Step® Plan, you are now ready for the maintenance diet. By boosting your daily total fat intake to between 25-30 grams of fat and your fiber intake to between 25-30 grams of fiber, you will be on the Diet-Step® Maintenance Diet. The maintenance diet varies with each individual, depending on height, weight, body build and your own individual metabolism. Some women can maintain their weight on 30 grams fat/30 grams fiber, while others will have to be content by staying on 25 grams fat/25 grams fiber to keep their weight off.

8. On this maintenance diet, you will keep all of the weight

off that you've already lost. You will not experience any of the rebound weight gain that is so common with most diet plans, particularly low carbohydrate diets. Rebound weight does not occur on the Diet-Step® Maintenance Plan, because by boosting dietary fiber to 25-30 grams daily, you in effect subdue the brain's hunger center (appestat). In other words, the more fiber you eat, the less weight you'll gain. Fiber fills you up without making you fat. The Diet-Step® Maintenance Plan will keep you trim and thin so that you can wear the smaller size clothes that you're now in.

9. If you notice that after you've been on the maintenance diet for a while and you start to gain a few pounds, then go back to the Quick Weight-Loss Diet-Step® Plan (20 Grams Fat/20 Grams Fiber) for a few weeks. After you're comfortably back into your clothes, you will have to find the right mix of fat and fiber (between 25-30 grams) that works for you. For example, you may find that you can maintain your weight on 25 grams of fat but you need 30 grams of fiber to control your appetite - then 25 grams of fat/30 grams of fiber is right for you. You can adjust the combination to fine-tune it for your own metabolism, based on how you look and feel. Your body will tell you the number of grams of fat and fiber that's right for you. Remember, the increased intake of fiber (fruits, vegetables, whole grains, legumes and beans) is what makes Diet-Step® work. Let fiber work for you, so that you don't have to work hard keeping the weight off.

10. Remember to eliminate all refined foods (sugar, flour and rice) and decrease the amount of salt, caffeine and alcohol from your diet. No more than (3) alcoholic drinks (wine or light beer) per week.

11.

    Enjoy at least 2-3 servings from the fruit group and 2-3 servings from the vegetable group each day. For a wide variety of nutrients, choose fruits and vegetables in a rainbow of colors. As you'll see in Chapter 3, these fruits and vegetables contain many disease fighting phyto-nutrients, vitamins and minerals which may reduce the risk of some cancers and help to prevent heart disease.

12. Choose from an array of high-fiber, nutritious, complex carbohydrates that fill you up without filling you out. These foods provide high-octane fuel to power you through the day and keep you energized for physical activity. The following foods are excellent sources of fiber: barley, oats, bran, wheat germ, bulgur and brown rice; beans, peas and lentils; whole-grain breads and pastas; and most fruits and vegetables including apples, broccoli, brussels sprouts, berries, cabbage, carrots, grapefruit, oranges, pears, plums, prunes, raisins and spinach, among others (see Fat & Fiber Counter in chapter 6).

13. Also remember to drink at least six 8 oz. glasses of water daily.

14. Don't forget to walk 20 minutes every day except Sunday or any other rest day that you choose. On the maintenance diet you only have to walk 5 days per week.

15. Now for the answer to the most important question you've been waiting for. "How much weight can I lose and how fast can I lose it on the Diet-Step®: 20 Grams/20 Minutes Plan?"

   a. You will lose approximately $2^1/_2$-3 pounds every week or 10-12 pounds for the 1st month.

   b. After the 1st month your weight loss will taper off to approximately $1^1/_2$-2 pounds per week as your body's metabolism adjusts to the 20 Grams Fat / 20 Grams Fiber Diet-Step® diet plan.

c. Need to lose weight even faster? No problem! Consult
Chapter 8 for even faster weight loss with the Fit-Step®
Plan.

20 GRAMS FAT/20 GRAMS FIBER
ALTERNATIVE MEAL PLANS

The following lists are a variety of 20 Grams Fat/20
Grams Fiber alternatives for your meal plans. Each meal
(breakfast, lunch & dinner) has already been pre-calculated
to add up to approximately 1/3 of the allotted fat and fiber
grams for each day. In other words, when you combine any
3 meals, you'll have the total allotted 20 grams fat/20 grams
fiber for any given day. Your bedtime snacks will be non-fat
with some fiber, so that for the sake of convenience, they
don't really have to be factored into the total grams of fat
and fiber each day. Actually, you'll probably be getting a
few more grams of fiber with your bedtime snacks.
Remember - Fiber Good! Fat Bad!

DIET-STEP®: BREAKFAST ALTERNATIVES

- 1 slice cinnamon french toast with egg substitute and
whole wheat bread
- 1 cup fat-free yogurt with fresh fruit and tblsp. wheat germ
- ½ cup low-fat granola with ½ cup blueberries and
strawberries
- 1 non-fat waffle with fresh fruit topping
- 1 toasted small whole wheat bagel with 1 tsp. non-fat
cream cheese
- 1 cup cooked oatmeal or wheatena with cinnamon and ¼
cup raisins
- 1 cup cold bran-type or whole wheat cereal with ½ cup
any fresh fruit
- 1 poached egg with 1 slice whole wheat toast and 1 tsp.
all-fruit jam

- 1 fried egg with non-fat spray and 1 slice whole wheat bread and 1 tsp. all-fruit jam
- 1 scrambled egg with non-fat spray and oat bran or whole wheat English muffin with 1 tsp. all-fruit jelly
- 2 egg white or egg substitute omelet with 1 slice low-fat (skim milk) cheese, tomato, onions, green peppers, mushrooms (any or all)
- 1 scooped-out whole wheat bagel with 1 slice unsalted smoked salmon (nova lox), with non-fat cream cheese, tomato and onion
- 2 small whole wheat or buckwheat pancakes made with egg substitute topped with fresh fruit and/or sugar free syrup
- 1 fried egg with non-fat spray and two small veggie non-fat sausages or two slices non-fat turkey bacon

DIET-STEP®: LUNCH ALTERNATIVES

- 1 veggie burger on whole wheat bread or bun with lettuce, tomato, onion & ketchup
- 1 tblsp. reduced-fat peanut butter & 1 tblsp. jelly sandwich whole wheat bread
- 2 tblsp. non-fat cream cheese sandwich on whole wheat bread with sprouts, tomato, cucumber and lettuce
- 1 non-fat cream cheese (2 tblsp.) and jelly (2 tblsp.) sandwich on whole wheat bread
- 1 medium whole wheat pita pocket with tuna (3 oz) packed in water with lettuce, tomato cucumber, sprouts and 1 tsp. Dijon mustard or 1 tsp. non-fat mayonnaise
- 1 medium whole wheat pita pocket with grilled chicken breast (3 oz) and 1 tsp. non-fat mayonnaise with lettuce, tomato, celery and cucumber
- 1 whole wheat sandwich with two slices skim milk cheese (alpine lace) or other low-fat cheese, with lettuce, tomato, shredded carrots and sprouts, with mustard or 1 tsp. non-fat mayonnaise
- 1 whole-wheat bun with two slices reduced-fat turkey breast, with lettuce, tomato, mustard or 1 tsp non-fat mayonnaise

- 1 cup soup (minestrone, lentil, split pea or any vegetable or bean-based soup) with one small whole-wheat roll
- 1 soft corn tortilla with 1/3 cup fat-free refried beans with shredded low-fat cheese, lettuce, tomato and salsa
- 1 medium order steamed mussels or clams (12) with ½ cup marinara sauce with 1 small whole wheat roll
- chicken caesar salad with lettuce, tomato, chopped celery, cucumber and with 3 oz grilled chicken breast and non-fat parmesan cheese and 1 tblsp. fat-free caesar dressing
- ½ veggie hoagie (tomatoes, lettuce, olives, peppers, onions, cucumbers, carrots, sprouts-your choice) with roll scooped out leaving only shell of Italian roll
- 1 whole-wheat bagel scooped out with one slice smoked salmon (nova lox) with tomato, onion and lettuce
- 1 whole-wheat bagel scooped out with 2 slices low-fat cheese, grilled with tomato and Dijon mustard or 1 tsp non-fat mayonnaise
- 1 can (3 oz) sardines (drain oil) on whole wheat bread or pita with tomato, lettuce and onion
- 1 slice pizza (tomato, or with light cheese and tomato) topped with veggies of your choice and a side salad with 1 tsp non-fat dressing
- Nicoise salad with mixed greens, tuna, string beans, tomato, anchovies, ½ sliced hardboiled egg, olives, radishes, celery, onions and bell pepper with mustard vinaigrette dressing on on the side (dip fork in dressing sparingly) and one scooped out French roll
- goat cheese salad with reduced-fat goat cheese, mixed greens, tomato, olives, bell peppers, cucumber, celery, with mustard vinaigrette dressing on the side (dip fork in dressing sparingly) and one scooped-out french roll
- panini sandwich toasted on scooped-out italian or french roll with tomato, low-fat mozzarella cheese, basil and lettuce
- spinach salad with 1 oz low-fat blue cheese, ½ oz. chopped walnuts, sliced apples, cherry tomatoes, cucumbers, in1 tblsp. dressing made with mustard, lemon and 1 tsp olive oil

DIET-STEP®: DINNER ALTERNATIVES

- 1 grilled 3 oz. lean hamburger on whole wheat roll with lettuce, tomato, onion and ketchup and 1 small white potato made into oven-baked french fries (slice into fries, spray nonstick pan with non-fat spray and bake on 400 degrees until crisp)
- 1 small can fat-free baked beans, 1 non-fat beef hot dog or turkey dog on whole wheat bun with sauerkraut, relish and mustard and small side salad with 1 tsp non-fat dressing
- 1 small can of sardines (drain oil) or tuna packed in water in large tossed salad of lettuce or romaine, tomato, cucumber, pepper, onion, sprouts, carrots and olives and 1 tsp non-fat dressing or mustard-vinaigrette dressing
- 1 cup spinach fettuccini with fresh vegetables and ½ cup tomato or marinara sauce and large tossed salad (see above)
- 1 cup whole wheat spaghetti with 12 clams or mussels, garlic, 1/3 cup white wine, 1 tsp olive oil and seasoning and large tossed salad (see above)
- 3 oz. grilled salmon steak or salmon fillet with tomatoes, onions, peppers and garlic and small baked potato or yam and 1 cup steamed vegetable (your choice)
- 1 cup Chinese greens with 6 medium grilled shrimp and garlic with 1 cup brown rice
- 2 soft tacos with non-fat refried beans, lettuce, tomato, onion, grated non-fat cheese with 3 oz. sliced grilled chicken and salsa
- 3 oz. lean roast beef with horseradish and small baked potato or yam with skin, 1 cup steamed veggies and small whole wheat roll
- 6 medium cooked peeled shrimp with cocktail sauce and small ear of corn and 1 cup steamed asparagus, broccoli or spinach
- 3 oz. broiled or baked cod, halibut, mackerel or sole with grilled onions, peppers, mushrooms and tomatoes, with lemon, wine and seasonings, small whole wheat dinner roll and tossed salad (see above)
- 2 small lamb chops (trim fat) with 2 tsp. mint jelly and whole broiled tomato with 1 small baked sweet potato and tossed salad (see above)

- 1cup low-fat macaroni and cheese with 1cup zucchini, diced tomatoes, onions and garlic and an ear of corn or a small sweet potato and steamed fresh carrots(½ cup)

YOUR OWN INDIVIDUAL DIET-STEP® PLAN

When you start to formulate your own combinations of 20 grams fat/20 grams fiber, you should keep a daily record of the total grams of fat and the total grams of fiber that you eat at each meal. Make sure that the total for each day adds up to no more than 20 grams fat and no less than 20 grams fiber. Use 3 x 5 index cards to keep your record for each individual meal. After you've recorded your meals each day, store the cards in a 3 x 5 index box divided into (4) sections: breakfast, lunch, supper, and snacks. Or, if you like, record the meals on different colored 3x5 index cards, for example: Yellow - breakfast (sunshine); Green - lunch (salads); Red - supper (hearty); and Blue -snack bedtime (calming). *Make it fun!* Then you can thumb through your cards at a later date to look up any meal that you'd like to have without having to add up the fat and fiber grams again. You'll end up with your own individual deck of 20 Grams Fat/20 Grams Fiber index cards, which will include all of the meal plans that you like the best. You can always add new and exciting recipes to your cards. For the computer-oriented woman on the go, you can record your meal plans on one of the many hand-held organizers or palm-type computers. Choose any method that's easy and fun for you.

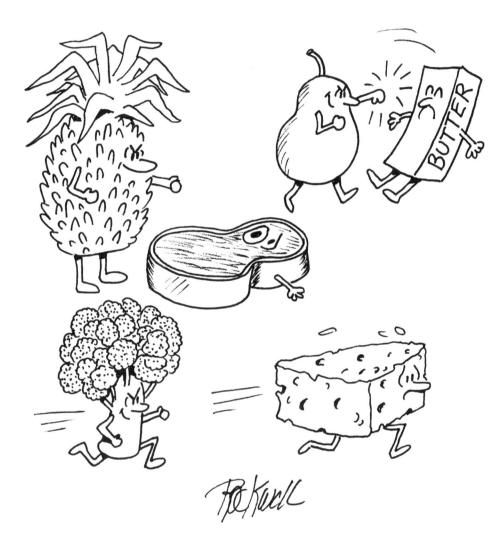

CHAPTER 3

FEARLESS FIBER: HEALTH POWER-HOUSE!
****

Fiber is the general term for those parts of <u>plant food</u> that we are unable to digest; however, bacteria present in the colon partly digests fiber through a process known as fermentation. Fiber is not found in foods of animal origin (meats and dairy products).

TYPES OF FIBER

Plant foods contain a mixture of different types of fibers. These fibers can be divided into soluble or insoluble depending on their solubility in water.

1. <u>Insoluble fibers</u>: (cellulose, hemi-celluloses, lignin) make up the structural parts of the cell walls of plants. These fibers absorb many times their own weight in water, creating a soft bulk to the stool and hasten the passage of waste products out of the body. These insoluble fibers promote bowel regularity and aid in the prevention and treatment of some forms of constipation, hemorrhoids, and diverticulitis. These fibers also may decrease the risk of colon cancer by diluting potentially harmful substances that are present in the colon.

2. <u>Soluble fibers</u>: (gums, pectins, and mucilages) are found within the plant cells. These fibers form a gel, which slows both stomach emptying and absorption of simple sugars from the intestines. This process helps to regulate blood sugar levels, which is particularly helpful in diabetic patients and is helpful in controlling weight in non-diabetics. Many soluble fibers can also assist in lowering blood cholesterol by binding with bile acids and cholesterol and eliminating the cholesterol through the

intestinal tract before the cholesterol can be absorbed into the blood stream.

Weight control is aided by the slower emptying of the stomach when you ingest soluble fibers. This causes a feeling of fullness and a decrease in hunger, causing fewer calories to be consumed. For example, if you eat an apple, which has a high fiber content, you'll have a feeling of fullness, as compared to eating a cupcake, which has no fiber, and which is the same weight and size as the apple. In fact, it would take approximately three cupcakes to satisfy your brain's hunger center before you realized that you were full. Well, by then you would already have consumed 480 calories and 16.5 grams of fat. The best sources of soluble fiber are fruits and vegetables, oat bran, barley, dried peas and beans, flax seed and psyllium.

3. Resistant starch: Approximately 15% of the starch in foods is tightly bound to fiber and resists the normal digestive processes. Bacteria normally present in the colon ferment this resistant starch and change it into short-chain fatty acids, which are important to normal bowel health and may also help to protect the colon from cancer-causing agents. Foods that contain resistant starch include breads, cereals, pasta, rice, potatoes and legumes.

HOW FIBER HELPS YOU LOSE WEIGHT

1. Fiber helps in weight loss and weight control by the simple fact that high-fiber foods contain fewer calories for their large volume. Fiber-rich foods, such as fruits and vegetables, whole grain cereals and breads, potatoes and legumes are low in fat calories and have a high water content. You are, therefore, eating less and enjoying it more.

2. High fiber foods have a high bulk ratio, which satisfies the hunger center more quickly than low fiber foods; consequently,

fewer calories are consumed. Fiber-rich foods take longer to chew and to digest than fiber-depleted foods, which, in turn gives your stomach time to feel full. Feeling full earlier leads to consuming fewer calories.

3. Foods with a <u>low-fiber</u> content are, in most cases, considerably <u>more concentrated in calories.</u> These fiber-deficient foods (fats, refined sugars, flour and alcohol) require hardly any chewing and have little or no bulk content. Therefore, large amounts of calories are consumed when eating these foods before your appetite center in the brain (appestat) is satisfied. These low-fiber foods are more concentrated in calories, so that more food must be eaten before the stomach can be filled.

4. <u>Removing fiber from food,</u> such as refining grains or flours (white bread, white rice, pasta, cereal) or by extracting the juices out of whole fruits (example: apple juice) and vegetables, results in the following negative features:

   a. High-fiber foods turn into <u>low-fiber foods.</u>
   b. Low-calorie foods turn into <u>high-calorie foods.</u>
   c. High-bulk foods turn into <u>low-bulk foods.</u>
   d. Longer eating time changes into shorter eating time, which <u>consumes more calories.</u>
   e. Easily satisfied hunger changes into <u>hunger not easily satisfied.</u>
   f. Complex carbohydrates slowly absorbed change into <u>simple sugars, which are quickly absorbed.</u>
   g. Slow absorption of food causes less insulin to be produced, which changes to <u>increased insulin production with subse-quent weight gain.</u>

FIBER-UP YOUR DIET

1. Drink 6-8 glasses of water daily. Fiber can absorb many times its own weight of water, providing bulk to the diet and a subsequent feeling of fullness.

2. Eat high-fiber whole grain cereals for breakfast, preferably those with 5 or more grams of fiber per serving. You can beef up the fiber content of cereals by adding 1½ tablespoons of unprocessed bran or wheat germ, if necessary.

3. Eat fresh fruit with skin, rather than fruit juices, which have little or no fiber content.

4. Use whole grain or fiber-enriched breads, which have more than double the fiber content of white bread.

5. Consume more vegetables, legumes and salads (without the dressing, of course, unless you use a little olive oil and vinegar). Include carrots, celery, cabbage, peas, broccoli, brussels sprouts, lentils, potatoes with skin, dried beans and baked beans (without sugar or bacon).

6. Snack foods should include dried fruits, nuts, seeds, high-fiber low-fat (1.5 grams total fat or less), snack bars, popcorn, celery and carrot sticks.

7. Add bran, nuts, seeds or grits to soups, yogurt or casseroles.

8. Use whole grain flour or soy flour instead of refined white flour. Eat whole grain pastas in place of regular pasta.

9. Use whole grain products (bran and whole grain cereals, brown long grain rice, and whole grain noodles).

10. Substitute whole grain bread (stone ground or whole wheat) or fiber enriched bread and bran instead of white refined breads.

11. Add garden vegetables (carrots, celery, cabbage, green beans, lettuce, onions, corn, peas, tomatoes, spinach, etc.).

12. Increase fruits (apples, oranges, pears, bananas, strawberries, blueberries, plums, peaches and cherries).

13. Legumes, seeds, nuts and beans are useful additions to a high fiber diet.

14. Unprocessed bran or wheat germ are dry bran/wheat powders, which are convenient high dietary fibers. Each level teaspoon contains two grams of dietary fiber. Either may be sprinkled on cereal or other foods, or it may be mixed in with orange or tomato juice to improve its taste.

15. Breads must have the word "whole" as the first listed ingredient

on the package, otherwise it's not a true whole-grain product, no matter how the bread is labeled.

A high-fiber diet is essentially a healthy, low-fat diet, which decreases the intake of refined foods. This encourages the consumption of fresh fruits, vegetables, whole grain cereals and breads. When the fiber is eaten from a variety of food sources, it produces its most beneficial effect, especially when it is eaten with each meal of the day.

Dietary fiber takes longer to chew and eat with the subsequent development of more saliva and a larger bulk swallowed with each mouthful. The larger bulk helps to fill the stomach and causes a decrease in hunger before more calories are consumed. High fiber diets help to provide bulk without energy, and may reduce the amount of energy absorbed from the food that is eaten. These high fiber diets are often referred to as having a low-energy density and appear to prevent excessive caloric (energy) intake. Countries that consume high fiber diets rarely have obesity problems.

COLORFUL FRUITS AND VEGETABLES: NOT JUST A PRETTY FACE

It is well documented that colorful fruits and vegetables contain cancer-fighting substances and offer a full spectrum of disease prevention. For maximum health benefits, you should eat a variety of vegetables and fruits of different colors (plant pigments). The reason for the different colors is that each colored fruit or vegetable has a different phyto-chemical (phyto means plant). These phyto-chemicals in the fruits and vegetables tend to decrease the risk of certain types of cancer. It is important to eat at least 4-5 servings of fruit or vegetables per day. The following is a list of some of the phyto-chemicals present in fruits and vegetables that can reduce your risk of cancer and heart disease:

1. Lycopene

   Lycopene is what gives many fruits and vegetables, including tomatoes, their deep red color. Lycopene is a carotenoid, or plant pigment, in the same family as beta-carotene. However, lycopene is not just a colorful addition to the fruit. Lycopene has powerful antioxidant properties that have been shown to fight different forms of cancer. National studies have shown that fruits and vegetables that contain lycopene, particularly tomatoes, may help to prevent prostate cancer, as well as colon, stomach, lung, esophageal and pancreatic cancers, according to the American Institute for Cancer Research. Lycopene has also been linked with a lower risk of heart attacks secondary to coronary artery disease.

2. Beta-carotene

   Beta-carotene is a powerful antioxidant, which has cancer-fighting properties. For example, sweet potatoes, which are high in dietary fiber, are loaded with cancer-fighting antioxidants (beta-carotene) and vitamins C and E. Other sources of beta-carotene are dark green leafy vegetables, such as spinach, kale, bok choy and other greens. Orange and deep yellow fruits and vegetables also have considerable amounts of beta-carotene: for example, pumpkins, winter squash, carrots, and cantaloupe.

3. Flavinoids

   Flavinoids are a group of phyto-chemicals found in many fruits, vegetables and grains. The type of flavinoid which is found in grapes is called resveratrol. This compound is found primarily in the skin of grapes. It is also present in grape juice and red wine. Several studies have shown that this type of flavinoid has been instrumental in fighting cancer of the colon, liver and breast. Resveratrol inhibits that growth of cancer by preventing the start of DNA damage in a cell and the transformation of a normal cell into a cancerous cell. It also helps to inhibit the growth and spread of tumor cells. Resveratrol also seems to be cardio-protective according to recent medical research.

4. Ellagic Acid
This phyto-chemical is present in many types of fruits, vegetables and grains. It appears to reduce the damage to DNA caused by carcinogens, such as tobacco smoke and air pollution. Berries contain high amounts of ellagic acid and it has been shown that as little as a cup of raspberries or blueberries slowed the growth of abnormal colon cells in humans, and, in some cases, prevented or destroyed the development of cells that were infected with the human papilloma virus (HPV), which is the cause of cervical cancer. This particular cancer-fighting agent has also been demonstrated to have similar effects on the cancer cells of the breast and pancreas.

5. Combinations of Antioxidants and Vitamins
Various berries, including strawberries, raspberries and blueberries, are packed with major antioxidants, carotenoids and vitamin C. These antioxidants are believed to counteract the formation of many chemical processes that contribute to the formation of cancer.

6. Allium Family
Certain plants contain compounds known as allyl sulfides, which are instrumental in activating enzymes in the body that break down certain cancer-causing substances. These cancer-fighting agents increase the body's ability to excrete the cancer-causing agents. Examples of the allium family include garlic, onions, shallots and leeks. There are many studies that have shown that people who eat lots of garlic have less cancer of the stomach and colon. It is thought that garlic blocks the growth of new cancer cells.

7. Cruciferous Vegetables
These vegetables are four-petaled flowers, which resemble

crosses. Vegetables in this group include broccoli, cabbage and cauliflower. These cruciferous vegetables, particularly broccoli, appear to protect the body against many types of cancer. Many studies have shown that people who eat an abundance of cruciferous vegetables have a reduced incidence of many types of cancers, including colon, bladder, prostrate, esophagus, lung, breast, cervix and larynx.

8. Anthocyanins
These are plant pigments that help to protect you from heart disease. They are present in cherries, purple grapes and purple grape juice, raspberries and strawberries.

9. Carotenoids
These compounds are antioxidant plant pigments that are converted to vitamin A by the body. There are several types: Beta-carotene is a major source of vitamin A, which lowers the risk for heart disease and certain types of cancer; lutein and zeaxanthin are carotenoids, which are linked to a reduced risk of age-related macular degeneration, a major cause of blindness in older individuals. Important sources of beta-carotene include apricots, cantaloupe, mangoes, papayas, carrots, sweet potatoes and dark green leafy vegetables. Important sources of lutein and zeaxanthin are green beans, greens (collard, kale, mustard, turnip), romaine and other dark lettuces, seaweed, spinach, squash (winter types and butternut).

10. Isoflavones
These compounds act as weak estrogens (phyto-estrogens). Eating approximately 100 milligrams of Isoflavones daily can improve bone density. Good sources of Isoflavones are soy milk, soy protein, tofu and textured vegetable proteins.

11. Indoles
Indoles are compounds that help to fight cancer. Good examples of foods with indoles are broccoli sprouts, brussels sprouts,

cabbage and cauliflower.

12. Folic Acid

This B vitamin helps prevent birth defects and lowers levels of homocysteine, which is an amino acid linked to heart disease. Excellent sources of folic acid include oranges, orange juice, broccoli, romaine and other dark lettuces, and spinach.

So, you can see that fiber is not just another pretty face. It is a face of multiple colors wherein each fruit and vegetable has its own individual face derived from its own plant pigment. Each one of these colorful fruits and vegetables offer a full spectrum of disease prevention.

DISORDERS RESULTING FROM LACK OF FIBER

1. **CONSTIPATION:** Constipation results from the delayed passage of stool material which is entirely due to the excess absorption of water from the large bowel. This, in turn, causes a dry, hard stool, which has a delayed passage through the intestinal tract. By preventing excess absorption of water from the bowel, dietary fiber increases the passage of a bulky soft stool with a more rapid transit through the intestinal tract. By world standards, Americans are almost universally constipated.

2. **DIVERTICULAR DISEASE OF THE COLON:** Diverticular disease or diverticulosis of the colon is thought to be caused by an increased pressure inside the colon, which results from the muscular effort that is necessary to move the stool along the colon. Abnormally high pressures caused by the lack of dietary fiber and constipation forces small pouches in the lining wall of the large intestine. These are referred to as diverticula or small pockets in the muscular wall of the large intestine. When these pockets become blocked-up, they can become infected. This results in a more serious disorder called diverticulitis

3. **APPENDICITIS:** While only in the investigational stage at this point, many investigators feel that acute appendicitis is a result of a diet low in dietary fiber. This results from excessive muscle contraction in the appendix wall and a blockage in the appendix by hard, fecal material, both of which result from inadequate dietary fiber.

4. **HIATAL HERNIA:** Hiatal hernia is defined as an upper protrusion of the top of the stomach through the diaphragm into the upper chest cavity. Constipation not only increases the pressure within the bowel itself but also within the abdomen during the straining at stool. These increased pressures are believed to force the junction of the esophagus and stomach upward into the chest cavity.

5. **CANCER OF THE COLON:** Some people seem to have an excessive amount of bile acids in the colon, on which bacteria may act to produce cancer producing agents, in particular nitrates or nitrosamines. The current theory is that an increased amount of dietary fiber will produce a large fecal volume, which will dilute these carcinogens and make their transit more rapid through the bowel, thus giving them less time to adhere or stick to the bowel wall and exert their cancer producing effects. A recent study indicated that there was no link to cereal grain dietary fiber and colon cancer. Other studies have refuted these findings and have stated that a combination of all types of fiber (fruits, vegetables and whole grains) does indeed help to prevent colon cancer.

6. **HEMORRHOIDS:** Hemorrhoids are thought to be caused by the increased intra-abdominal pressure transmitted from the abdominal veins during straining at stool to the anal veins. Constipation resulting from a lack of dietary fiber also produces a shearing stress when passing hard stools, causing the attachments of the anal veins to become stretched. Rectal hemorrhoids plague one out of every two Americans over the age of

50. In England, patients with hemorrhoids are almost never referred to surgeons, but are routinely treated with high fiber diets.

7. **GALLSTONES:** Gallstones occasionally result from bile which is overloaded with a crystalloid type of cholesterol. There is evidence that dietary fiber reduces this type of cholesterol and increases the more beneficial components of the bile, thus reducing the tendency toward stone formation.

8. **DIABETES:** Low-carbohydrate diets are being replaced by diets higher in carbohydrates, particularly the complex starches or carbohydrates. Refined sugars are almost totally eliminated from this type of diet. Since this diet is higher in fiber, the intestinal content becomes more gelatinous (thicker) and subsequently slows the absorption of energy (and sugar) from the intestinal tract. This has a protective effect against the development of either high or low blood sugar levels after eating, since slow absorption produces an even distribution of sugar in the blood. In type 2 diabetes, fiber helps to regulate insulin production. Diabetes is rarely found in populations that consume high levels of dietary fiber.

9. **OBESITY:** High fiber foods such as fruits, vegetables, nuts and bran cereals generally require a longer time to eat since they require more chewing and tend to be bulky. This may help to create a feeling of fullness. With foods that are low in dietary fiber, more food is ingested before a sense of fullness has been attained. This low fiber food is usually eaten more rapidly, requires less chewing, is not bulky in character, and, therefore, enters the stomach more rapidly. Since it takes time for nerve impulses to reach the appetite control center, the feeling of hunger is not shut off until excessive amounts of low dietary fiber foods are eaten, and obesity is almost certain to result.

10. **VARICOSE VEINS:** There is strong evidence to indicate that

straining at stool caused by lack of dietary fiber increases the intra-abdominal pressure and these pressures are directly transmitted to the veins draining the leg. Repeated high pressures caused by straining enlarges these veins, stretching their small valves, which normally prevent the leakage of blood backwards in the veins. Since it is these valves which assist the upward flow of blood, their loss of function combined with gravity raises the pressure in the veins of the legs and results in varicose veins.

11. CORONARY HEART DISEASE: Dietary fiber binds with bile acids and cholesterol in the intestinal tract and subsequently reduces their absorption from the bowel into the blood stream. This may help to explain why in under-developed countries with a high proportion of dietary fiber there is a low prevalence of coronary heart disease. On a high fiber diet, studies show that blood fats were significantly reduced (cholesterol was reduced 25 percent and triglycerides 15 percent).

12. BREAST DISEASE: Recent studies have indicated that there may be a relationship between fiber intake and breast disease. This is based on the fact that substances which are potentially carcinogenic or contain excess female hormones may enter the blood stream from the colon and reach the breast tissue. These substances may then have a stimulating effect by producing either benign cystic breast disease and possibly cancer of the breast tissue. Dietary fiber may possibly play an indirect role in the prevention of these disorders by preventing or decreasing the absorption of these substances or hormones.

FIBER FIGHTS HEART DISEASE IN WOMEN

New findings from the Nurses' Health Study in 1998/1999, shows that fiber, especially cereal products, protects against heart disease. This study examined the relationship between fiber consumption as reported by nearly 70,000 women from 1984 through

1998. Women who ate an average of 23 grams of fiber a day had a 47% lower risk of major coronary events including myocardial infarction, and/or fatal coronary heart disease compared to those who ate about half as much fiber. When the researchers analyzed the individual effects of three different fiber sources (fruits, vegetables and cereals), only cereal fiber significantly reduced the risk of cardiovascular disease. A daily bowl of cold whole-grain breakfast cereal that supplies 5 or more grams of fiber cut heart disease risk by approximately 37%. This study was reported in the Journal of the American Medical Association in 1999. In this particular study of 70,000 women by the Nurses' Health Study, the ages of the women ranged from 37 to 64 years of age. None of the women in this study had a previous diagnosis of heart disease, stroke, cancer, diabetes or high cholesterol. It is proposed that the increased consumption of whole grain products may increase insulin sensitivity and lower triglyceride levels. Also, whole grain products including cereals are important sources of phyto-estrogens and may favorably affect blood coagulation activity (JAMA, October 27, 1999, volume 282, number 16.).

FRUIT AND VEGETABLES REDUCE THE RISK OF STROKE

The nutrients in fruits and vegetables, such as dietary fiber and antioxidants, are associated with a lower risk of heart disease, but few studies have examined their relationship to the risk for stroke. This study, reported in the Journal of the American Medical Association described the association between fruit and vegetable intake and ischemic stroke in over 75,000 women enrolled in the Nurses' Health Study and 38,000 men in the health professional follow-up study. Everyone in this particular study had no history of cardiovascular disease, stroke, cancer, diabetes or high cholesterol. During the follow-up period, which included fourteen years for women, and eight years for men, each increment of one serving of fruit or vegetables per day was associated with a seven percent reduction for risk of ischemic stroke in women, and a four percent reduction in men. This would translate into a *35% reduction in stroke for women* who ate five servings daily of fruit and vegetables. This study showed that there was no further reduction in the risk of stroke above 5 - 6 servings of fruit and vegetables per day. The consumption of a variety of vegetables and fruits, such as cruciferous vegetables (examples: broccoli and cabbage), green leafy vegetables, citrus fruits or vitamin - C rich fruits and vegetables resulted in the largest decrease in risk. Pretty impressive results for sticking to your high fiber diet of fruits and veggies (<u>JAMA</u> 1999, October 6, Volume 282, number 13).

INCREASED FIBER INTAKE CORRELATES WITH DECREASED MORTALITY FROM ALL CAUSES

In a recent study, in the <u>American</u> <u>Journal</u> <u>of</u> <u>Epidemiology</u>, women on a high fiber diet showed a significantly reduced risk from coronary heart disease and death from all causes. This study reviewed dietary data from the Scottish Heart Study on approximately 12,000 women and men ages 40 to 59 years of age. Women with a high intake of fiber had the greatest reduced risk of mortality from all causes, including coronary heart disease. These results suggest that the current public health drive to increase vitamin and fiber intake to at least five portions of fruit and vegetables a day should have beneficial effects on all causes of mortality.

These researchers attributed the beneficial effects of fiber to the fact that folate, the antioxidant active flavinoids, and minerals (selenium, magnesium and copper) will be co-ingested at higher levels in high-fiber, fruit and vegetable-rich diets. In addition, the stool-bulking properties of fiber may play an important role. Along with fiber, the study participants ingested other compounds present in fruits and vegetables that may have an added effect on the prevention of coronary heart disease and on all types of mortality. The antioxidant vitamin E showed the strongest beneficial effect with vitamin-C and beta-carotene. This study also showed that consuming high levels of fiber and antioxidants were associated with significantly lower rates of coronary heart disease and all types of mortality in a greater degree in women than in men (<u>American Journal of Epidemiology, 1999, 150: 1073- 1080</u>).

SPINACH: THE HEALTH POWERHOUSE

If you're looking for a vegetable with super healing powers, try spinach. It's packed with vitamins, antioxidants and minerals that will protect you from many diseases. Spinach contains many antioxidants including beta and alpha carotenes, lutein, zeaxanthin, potassium, magnesium, vitamin K and folic acid. Recent studies at two major universities have found that, as strange as it seems, spinach may lower the risk of strokes, colon cancer, cataracts, heart disease, osteoporosis, hip fractures, memory loss, Alzheimer's disease, depression and even birth defects. The disease fighting properties in spinach are better absorbed when spinach is cooked with a little olive oil. Now, that's what I call a super, super vegetable.

FIBER AND FIBROIDS

Benign uterine fibroids are the most commonly diagnosed uterine tumors. They have been associated with anemia, pelvic pain and, in some cases, fertility problems. It appears that women who have high levels of estrogens, which may be related to high meat intake, are more prone to fibroids. A recent study showed that diets decreasing or eliminating meats and increasing green vegetables have a significant effect on the prevention of the development of fibroids. The vegetables and fruits contain iso-flavinoids, which can offset the effect of estrogen on the body. Also, by eliminating meat from the diet, the levels of estrogen in the body decrease. By decreasing meat and increasing fiber, the body is less likely to develop estrogen related uterine fibroid tumors.

FIBER K.O.'S HEART DISEASE

In a recent study in the <u>American Journal of Clinical Nutrition,</u> women who ate three to four servings of whole grains a day had 1/3 to 1/2 the risk of developing heart disease as opposed to women who ate refined flour, such as white bread. It is important to check the ingredients in any commercial food to see that it is truly made from whole grains. In particular, it is important to check the ingredients in snack foods (for example; cookies, crackers and chips), since many of these products contain not only refined white flour, but also partially hydrogenated oils (trans-fats), which actually can raise your cholesterol more than other types of saturated fats.

FLAWED FIBER STUDY

In January 1999, a group of Boston researchers reported no difference in the rates of colon or rectal cancer in women who ate a high fiber diet as opposed to those who ate a low fiber diet. This study was eventually refuted by qualified researchers who pointed out that, in this particular study, the only type of fiber that was studied was cereal fiber. Women, for example, metabolize fiber differently from men. Female hormones and hormone replacement therapy after menopause also helped protect against colon cancer in many cases, as they do against heart disease. Moreover, with so many different kinds of fiber included in a healthy diet, the evidence of scientific studies on the impact of plant foods and their fiber is still in its infancy. Recent studies have subsequently shown that high fiber diets, which include not only cereal grains, but fruits and vegetables, do, indeed, help to prevent against the development of colon cancer. As part of the on-going Nurses' Health Study that provided the data questioning the preventive role of fiber, a 1998 report showed that women who ate a diet high in red meat had higher rates of colorectal cancer. In that same study, women whose diets were low in red meat and high in fruits, vegetables and cereal grains had a significantly decreased risk of colon cancer. In countries where diets are high in plant-based foods and low in red meat and animal fat, people have lower rates of heart disease and colon cancer.

BLUEBERRIES MAY REVERSE AGING PROCESS

New research has indicated that women on antioxidant-rich diets showed fewer age-related disorders than those on a normal diet. The studies showed that among all the fruits and vegetables, the benefits were greatest with blueberries, which reversed age-related effects, for example: loss of balance and lack of coordination. They also discovered that blueberry extract had the greatest effect on reversing aging decline. Antioxidants help neutralize free radical by-products on the conversion of oxygen into energy, which, if not neutralized, can cause oxidative stress and lead to cell damage. Previous studies have shown that both strawberries and spinach extract can also help to prevent the onset of age-related defects. However, the greatest effect was shown in patients who ate blueberries; phyto-nutrients in blueberries, particularly flavinoids and beta-carotene seem to have an anti-inflammatory effect, which may even help in the prevention of Alzheimer's disease. Again, we have another solid recommendation for eating fruits and vegetables because of their high fiber content and because of their phyto-nutrient and antioxidant powers (The Journal of Neuroscience, September 15, 1999; 19: 8114-8 1 21).

THE FRENCH PARADOX

There are three known factors contributing to atherosclerosis (hardening of the arteries):

1. Overactive platelet activity, which causes blood to stick and can lead to a heart attack or stroke.
2. High levels of LDL (bad) cholestero1. Free radicals can oxidize LDL cholesterol and contribute to the build-up of plaque in the arteries.
3. The third contributing factor to atherosclerosis is damage to endothelial cells.

Patients on a diet high in purple grapes had an almost tripling of the blood vessels' ability to respond to the increased blood flow, and also showed a slower onset of LDL oxidation, meaning that it is less likely that the oxidation will contribute to atherosclerosis. The flavinoid (trans-resveratrol) in purple grapes is the key to the prevention of atherosclerosis. Fruits, vegetables, nuts, and seeds also contain flavinoids, as well as red wine. This research is often referred to as the French Paradox, which helps to explain the low incidence of heart disease in France, where red wine consumption is high. While people in France eat almost three times as much saturated fat as Americans, the French have only 1/3 the risk of heart disease. The same heart disease prevention benefits appear to be related to the consumption of purple grapes, which contain the same flavinoids as red wine (Circulation October 1999, 100: *1050-1055*).

VEGGIES DECREASE RISK OF BLADDER CANCER

In a recent study on bladder cancer, it was shown that in order to reduce the risk of bladder cancer, it is necessary to drink lots of fluids, not to smoke and to eat lots of cruciferous vegetables. A high intake of cruciferous vegetables, particularly broccoli and cabbage, significantly reduced the risk of bladder cancer. This may be explained by the presence of one or more phyto-chemicals in broccoli and cabbage, which are specific in the reduction of bladder cancer risk. This study also showed that a high intake of fruits, yellow vegetables and green leafy vegetables did not significantly reduce the risk of bladder cancer. The relationship with high cruciferous vegetable intake (broccoli and cabbage) were associated with the highest reduction in the risk of developing bladder cancer (Journal National Cancer Institute, 1999; 91 (no. 7): 605-613).

ORANGES PROTECT YOUR HEART AND FIGHT CANCER

In a recent study, it was shown that oranges boost HDL cholesterol in addition to providing vitamin-C, folic acid and numerous flavinoids. These compounds are thought to prevent cholesterol oxidation, which has been linked to a reduced risk of coronary events.

An orange or two a day will keep atherosclerosis away. Researchers have found that citrus fruits, in particular oranges, also showed anti-cancer activity in animals and in test tubes. These researchers found that animals that drank orange juice for several months were 25% less likely to develop early colon cancer than animals given only water. Compounds such as liminoids in orange juice seem to alter the characteristics of the colon lining, discouraging cancer growth. These researchers also speculate that the orange juice may also help to suppress breast, prostrate and lung cancer (Circulation, 100; 101: 1050-1055, 1999).

PROTECT YOUR EYESIGHT WITH VEGGIES

Kale and spinach are two vegetables rich in the antioxidants lutein and zeaxanthin. These antioxidants have been reported to protect against age related cataracts and macular degeneration, one of the leading causes of blindness. Also high in these vision-protecting antioxidants are romaine lettuce, broccoli, collards, turnip greens and corn.

FIBER HELPS PREVENT BREAST AND UTERINE CANCER

Women who limit their intake of red meat and eat lots of green vegetables have a reduced risk of developing breast cancer and uterine cancer. High levels of estrogen, which results from the consumption of beef, ham, pork and other red meat, have been implicated in the formation of breast and uterine cancer. The intake of 4 - 5 servings of fruits and vegetables daily with phyto-nutrients, in particular, iso-flavinoids, may offset some of estrogen's effect on the uterus and breast (Obstetrics and Gynecology, 94 [No. 3]: 395-398, 1999).

SOYBEANS: THE NEW FIBER HEALTH FOOD

Soybeans contain soy proteins, which helps to reduce the risk of cardiovascular disease. The reason for this is that soy proteins reduce the amount of total fat and LDL cholesterol in the blood by affecting the synthesis and metabolism of cholesterol in the liver. Its amino acid composition differs from the structure of other proteins found in meat and milk. Clinical trials showed a significantly lower incidence of coronary heart disease in patients with a high soy intake. Soybeans can be found in many different varieties, including soy beverages, tofu, tempeh, soy-based meat substitutes, and some baked goods. However, to qualify, such soy-rich foods should contain at least 6.5 grams of soy protein, and less than 3 grams of total fat per serving and less than 1 gram of saturated fat per serving in order to qualify as a heart health food.

In another related study, soy supplements were shown to cut the risk of developing colon cancer in half. Soy supplements also decreased the relative risk of having a recurrence of colon cancer in high-risk subjects. This study was reported at the annual conference of The American Institute for Cancer Research. High soy intake may be able to delay the onset of colon cancer in those at risk, or may lead to more cancer-free years in those whose initial cancer was surgically removed.

THE MEDITERRANEAN DIET

Research shows that the Mediterranean diet, which emphasizes whole grains, greens, fruits, vegetables, fish and olive oil, is healthier than the typical American diet, which is high in fat and processed foods. There is a significantly decreased risk of heart disease and cancer in the Mediterranean cultures, which have been thriving on these foods for thousands of years. The Mediterranean diet has been found to help protect against heart disease and help to control blood cholesterol and blood sugar levels. In the Mediterranean diet, people consume at least 20 to 25 grams of fiber a day. In addition to fiber, this diet is rich in *omega-3 fatty acids* from fish oils and *alpha-linoleic acid* from plant sources. Both of these substances help fiber to reduce the incidence of heart disease.

The Mediterranean diet can be explained quite simply by explaining what is actually whole grain. Grains consist of three layers: 1) the inner germ, 2) the middle endosperm, and 3) the outer bran. Processing white flour and white rice keeps the two inside layers, but removes the outside layer, the bran, with its fiber, vitamins and minerals. With whole grains, you get all of those nutrients plus complex carbohydrates, protein, fiber, antioxidants and phytochemicals that may help guard against cancer and heart disease. Also, whole grains provide energy and calories with little fat, and they can lengthen the time that it takes to digest foods, so that you feel full longer. This simple explanation of why the Mediterranean diet is far superior to our western diet, shows us why fiber is a significantly important factor in the Diet-Step® 20 Grams Fat/20 Grams Fiber Diet Plan.

THE TOP 20 ANTIOXIDANT FOODS

Fruits	**Veggies**	**Honorable mention**
Apples	Broccoli	Apricots
Blueberries	Bok Choy	Cantaloupe
Blackberries	Cabbage	Cauliflower
Cherries	Carrots	Greens (others)
Cranberries	Garlic	Mangoes
Prunes	Kale	Nuts
Purple Grapes	Spinach	Olive Oil
Raisins	Squash	Onions
Raspberries	Sweet potatoes	Tea
Strawberries	Tomatoes	Whole Grains

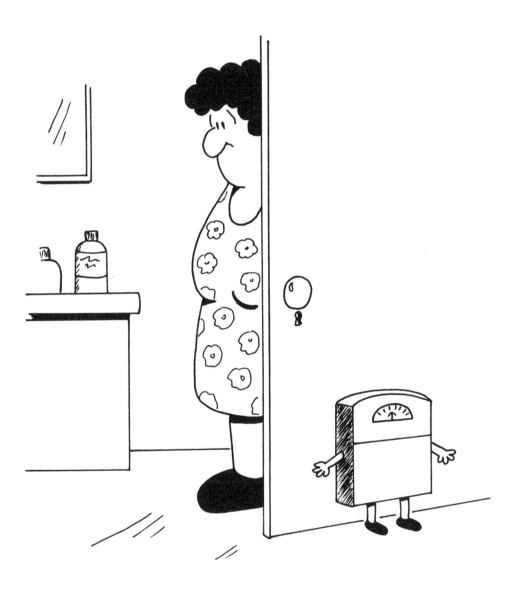

CHAPTER 4

FEARSOME FAT: BE VERY AFRAID!

****

FAT FACTS

In a study just released by the National Heart, Lung and Blood Institute in Bethesda, Maryland, obesity has now been listed as a major independent risk factor for heart disease. What's so new about that? Everyone knows that being overweight contributes to heart disease. That's just it; up until now obesity was just a contributing factor in heart disease because of its relationship with high blood pressure and high cholesterol. Now it has gained its own independent rating as causing heart disease all by itself. This study, consisting of 5,000 women and men, was followed for 26 years. The risk of developing heart disease was more pronounced in people who gained most of their excess weight after the age of 25.

In this study, obesity ranked third in men and fourth in women in predicting coronary heart disease. The other factors in heart disease were high blood pressure, serum cholesterol, cigarette smoking, age, diabetes and electrocardiogram abnormalities. Only high blood pressure, cholesterol and age were ranked ahead of obesity with cigarette smoking a close fourth in predicting heart disease. One important point made in this extensive study was: *losing a moderate amount of weight lessened the risk of developing heart disease.*

According to the American Heart Association, more than 41 million Americans have one or more forms of heart or blood vessel disease.

Heart attacks claimed 550,000 lives in 1999, 56 percent of all deaths from cardiovascular disease. The Heart Association estimated that as many as one million Americans will have a heart attack this year and more than one-third of them will die.

Stroke was listed as the second leading cause of death in cardiovascular disease, which claimed 185,000 lives in 1999. They estimated that 1.8 million Americans are survivors of stroke.

High Blood Pressure: one in every four adults or 35 million Americans suffer from high blood pressure. In 1999, over 175,000 people died from the complications of high blood pressure.

Cardiovascular disease accounts for more than 45 percent of all deaths that occur in the United States yearly, and in most cases, is caused by atherosclerosis. Since obesity is often associated with elevated blood cholesterol levels, it is thought to be indirectly responsible for the development of atherosclerosis (fat deposits in arteries). Recent studies also indicate that obesity also increases the risk of developing hypertension. In many mild cases of high blood pressure, weight loss alone can serve as an effective treatment. The following charts, "FACTS ABOUT FAT," will illustrate what happens inside your body as fat accumulates (Figs. 1 & 2).

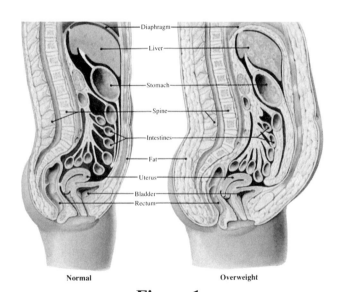

Normal   Overweight

Figure 1

Courtesy of Medical Times

Normal Amount of Fat

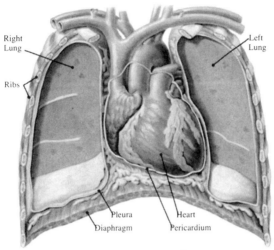

Right
Lung

Left
Lung

Ribs

Pleura   Heart
Diaphragm   Pericardium

Excess Amount of Fat

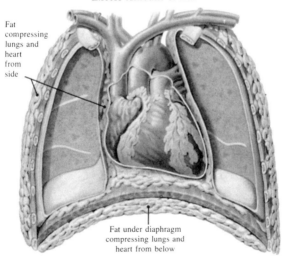

Fat
compressing
lungs and
heart
from
side

Fat under diaphragm
compressing lungs and
heart from below

Figure 2
Courtesy of Medical Times

Shortness of breath may be a first sign of pulmonary distress and heart strain caused by being overweight. The chart shows you how and why obesity increases the heart's workload and contributes to premature death: fat enlarges the capillary bed (tiny connective blood vessels in an area or organ of your body) which increases the amount of tissue to be nourished by the blood and through which the blood must be pumped by your heart.

In addition, the fat accumulated has to go someplace. You can see what's happening on the outside of you. Now, let's take a look at the inside. Fat infiltrates the liver and other organs. It's a squeeze process, an invasion. Fat compresses the heart, decreases the blood supply to the intestines, etc. (See figures above). Some very obese people can't sit, because if they do, there's no space for their lungs to operate in, as the fat invades the chest. These people have to stand up or lie down all the time. They have disabled themselves. Along with all this, extra heavy people, and even moderately overweight persons, are putting an extra burden on their backs and legs (the weight bearing joints), which causes or increases arthritic problems.

Complications following surgery occur more frequently in obese people. Wounds don't heal as well or as fast. And again, there is a breathing problem; overweight people can't take anesthesia as well as people of normal weight.

WEIGHT CONTROL BY CONTROLLING INTAKE OF FAT

Controlling our weight by reducing the amount of saturated fat and cholesterol in our diet has a two-fold benefit. First of all, it will help control and maintain our weight. Second, it will have a beneficial effect on the prevention of cardiovascular and cerebrovascular disease, since, as we have seen, these illnesses have been associated with high levels of blood cholesterol.

The typical *American diet* has a higher fat content than nearly any other country in the world. There is little doubt that this increased fat intake in our diet is responsible for the development of *obesity*, as well as many other disorders. Fat is the most concentrated source of calories, since a gram of dietary fat supplies your body with *nine calories.* This is compared to only four calories per gram of protein or carbohydrate. Since fat has this concentrated source of calories, it is the *most fattening* type of food that we consume and it stands to reason that cutting down on the fat intake is one of the best ways to cut down on the total amount of calories and to maintain normal body weight.

All foods that are of *plant origin* do not contain cholesterol. These include fruits, vegetables, grains, cereals, nuts, and vegetable oils (coconut and palm oil are the only exceptions). In choosing vegetable oils, make sure that you choose liquid monosaturated or polyunsaturated vegetable oils, rather than solid or hydrogenated vegetable oil products, since these liquid oils have a beneficial effect in helping to lower blood cholesterol. Recent studies have found that monosaturated fats are even more beneficial than polyunsaturated fats.

WHAT IS CHOLESTEROL?

Cholesterol is a *fat-like substance* normally found in all living tissue and is an essential chemical for health. It is found in every cell and fluid in the body. Although it resembles fat in many ways, it has a completely different chemical structure called steroid lipids. Cholesterol also differs from fat, in that it is not used by the body as food for the production of energy. Cholesterol is extremely important, however, in the *metabolism of fat* and the production of *hormones* in the body. It is equally important in the formation of *bile salts*, which aids in our digestion. *Cholesterol* also forms an important structural component of the *membranes* (walls) of all the body's cells.

Since the body requires a certain amount of cholesterol all the time, it is manufactured naturally in our bodies, primarily in the liver. So, what's the problem? It looks as if cholesterol is pretty good for our health. Well it is, providing there's not too much of it. Unfortunately, we also get cholesterol into our bodies in the food we eat and that is where the problem begins. Medical research has shown that when we take in *too much cholesterol* in our diets, the amount of cholesterol in our blood begins to rise. Once there is an excessive amount of cholesterol circulating in our blood stream, it starts to build up in the walls of the arteries. These yellow-rubbery deposits of cholesterol called *plaques* narrow the passageway of the artery (hardening of the arteries). This condition often leads to *heart attacks and strokes* since not enough blood can get through these narrowed blood vessels.

WHAT IS SATURATED FAT?

Saturated fat is present in all products of *animal origin*: meat, fish, fowl, eggs, butter, milk, cream and cheese. Saturated fats are also found in some *vegetable products,* which are usually solid or semi-solid at room temperature. They include *shortenings* and *table spreads* which have been changed from liquid fats (usually cottonseed and soybean oils) into solids by a process called *hydrogenation.* This process makes the products more suitable for table use and prevents them from becoming rancid. However, this process converts polyunsaturated fats into *saturated fats.*

Other saturated fats in the vegetable kingdom include *cocoa butter, palm oil and coconut oil.* Most people are unaware of the fact that they consume significant amounts of coconut **and** palm oil. It is used commercially in a wide variety of processed foods, baked goods and deep-fat fried products.

Saturated fats are dangerous because they can increase the amount of cholesterol in the blood. These fats can raise the level of blood *cholesterol* as much as, if not more than, the actual consumption of dietary cholesterol products. These fats can also interfere with brain function and can actually cause damage to the brain cells by interfering with the brain's circulation. This can lead to memory loss, difficulty concentrating, confusion and may even accelerate Alzheimer's disease.

There are five factors that can help to **lower your blood cholesterol** which we will be discussing in this chapter:

1. Decrease the total amount of fat in your diet
2. Decrease the amount of dietary cholesterol that you eat.
3. Decrease the amount of saturated fat in your diet.
4. Increase the amount of mono-saturated fats, and to a lesser extent, polyunsaturated fats in your diet.
5. Walk 20 minutes six days per week.

WHAT ARE UNSATURATED FATS?

1. **Monosaturated fats** (neutral fats) may actually help to increase the *good HDL cholesterol level,* and, therefore, they have been found to be cardio-protective. They are usually liquid at room temperature and tend to harden or cloud when refrigerated. They are the primary fats found in *olive oil, canola oil, peanut oil* and *most nuts.* They are also present in small amounts in meats, dairy products and some vegetables. These are *good fats.*

2. **Polyunsaturated fats** (essential fatty acids) are always of *vegetable origin* and are *liquid oils.* Safflower oil is the highest in polyunsaturates of all oils. Sunflower oil is second, followed by corn oil, sesame seed oil, soybean oil, cottonseed oil, walnut oil and linseed oil. Polyunsaturated fats may help to *lower the bad LDL cholesterol level* by assisting the body to eliminate excessive amounts of newly manufactured cholesterol.

It is essential that you substitute monounsaturated and polyunsaturated fats for saturated fats to maximize their cholesterol-lowering effect. It is interesting to note that we can manufacture saturated fat and most monosaturated fats in our bodies. Polyunsaturated fats must be obtained from the diet and are, therefore, *called essential fatty acids.* However, polyunsaturated vegetable oils, which are found in margarine, salad dressings, corn oil and processed foods, contain *omega-6 type fats.* These are also considered bad fats when excessive amounts are consumed, since they can set up chronic inflammation in brain tissue, which could lead to brain damage, strokes and degenerative brain diseases like Alzheimer's disease. Therefore, polyunsaturated oils should be limited to 1 ½ tsp. daily.

3. **Trans-fats** are partially hydrogenated oils and are *bad fats.* They can increase your risk of heart disease by raising your cholesterol. They are found in many baked foods, cookies, crackers, snack foods, etc. Always check food labels for *partially hydrogenated oils*, which are actually trans-fats. Avoid them.

WHAT ARE LIPIDS?

The term lipids is used to include *all fats and fat-like substances* (e.g., cholesterol). These lipids will not dissolve in water and are called *fat-soluble substances.* How do they get absorbed into the blood stream, since the blood is a water-soluble solution? These lipids (fats and cholesterol) hook up with certain proteins so that they can dissolve in water (in this case, the blood) and are now called **Lipo-Proteins**. The protein acts as the submarine, transporting its passenger, Mr. Fat or Mr. Cholesterol, through the blood stream.

There are several types of lipo-protein combinations present in our bodies; however, for our purposes we will discuss two of the most important ones.

1. The **Bad-Cholesterol-Submarine** (LDL-low density lipo-protein combination). This bad submarine (LDL) deposits cholesterol in your arteries when too much cholesterol is taken into the diet or manufactured by the body. You can help here *by eating less saturated fats and cholesterol-rich foods.* Consequently, the bad submarine will have less cholesterol to carry and therefore won't be able to clog up your arteries.

2. The **Good-Cholesterol-Submarine** (HDL-high density lipo-protein combination) is quite a different story. It acts opposite to the bad submarine, by collecting the excess amounts of cholesterol in the blood and taking it to the liver where it is eliminated from the body in the bile juices. Some medical investigators also feel that this good submarine (HDL) may be able to shovel the cholesterol out of the cholesterol deposits (plaques) that have already formed in your arteries in the early stages.

Well, how do we get some of this good HDL? As always, there's got to be a catch. First, heredity plays an important part in HDL production. Some of us have more than others because of good genes. There's nothing we can do about that. Secondly, diet plays almost no role in affecting HDL production, except for adding monosaturated fats to the diet, which can help to raise HDL. Smoking, incidentally, has been shown to lower HDL: another nail in its coffin. Many people who have elevated LDL (bad) cholesterol and low HDL (good) cholesterol because of hereditary factors often have to take cholesterol-lowering medications called Statins.

Fortunately, there is another thing that we can do **to help** raise HDL production in our bodies. Medical research has definitely shown that a regular program of a moderate intensity exercise -- **WALKING** -- can raise our HDL levels. This type of exercise must be continued on a regular basis in order to keep this HDL elevated. Short bursts of exercise (high intensity exercise, e.g., jogging) only temporarily raises the HDL level, which decreases abruptly after the exercise is stopped. The lifetime Diet-Step®/Fit-Step® plan is the **best** answer to this problem.

CHOLESTEROL AND ITS ASSOCIATION WITH HEART DISEASE

1. *Animal studies* show that when laboratory animals are put on a standard, high cholesterol American diet, they develop atherosclerosis or hardening of the coronary arteries. They have considerably less heart disease when they are placed on cholesterol lowering diets and/or medications to lower cholesterol.

2. *The Framingham Heart Study,* which has been in progress since 1958 and has followed over 5,000 people, has repeatedly shown that the blood cholesterol level is one of the strongest predictors of a person's risk for developing coronary heart disease. In this study, cholesterol is coupled with other risk factors such as blood pressure, smoking, family history, and lack of exercise.

3. In people who have *heart disease* at very young ages or in families where there is a high prevalence of heart disease, cholesterol levels are usually found to be high. Epidemiological studies comparing different nations and cultures show that populations who have a high fat intake have significantly more heart disease than cultures with less fat in their diets. In addition, when certain ethnic groups migrate to a new cultural society, they tend to develop both the cholesterol blood levels and risks of heart disease of their new environments. This suggests that environmental factors such as high cholesterol diets may be more crucial than genetic factors in determining the risk of developing heart disease.

4. The microscopic examination of the coronary arteries taken from autopsies shows that cholesterol is always present in the areas where the coronary arteries were blocked. Studies also indicate that this cholesterol found in these areas of blockage has moved into the vessel wall from the blood stream.

There appears to be little doubt from this evidence that the relationship of high levels of *blood cholesterol* to the development of *coronary heart disease* is a significant risk factor. The major factor in reducing the level of cholesterol in the blood is to reduce the amount of *total fat in the diet* (Diet-Step®: 20 Grams Fat/20 Grams Fiber Diet). This usually means switching from fatty meats and pork products to leaner meats, fish and poultry. Also, one should reduce the amount of dairy fat in the diet, switching from whole to skim milk and avoiding the use of butter and cream. Also, low-fat/skim milk cheeses are preferable to regular cheese.

A second important factor in determining the level of blood cholesterol is the *type of fat eaten.* Most animal fats are saturated fats, whereas most vegetable oils are *polyunsaturated fats.* Studies have shown that substituting polyunsaturated for saturated fats does result in lowering the blood cholesterol level, even if the total amount of fat in the diet is the same. *Monosaturated fats* may play an even more important role in the prevention of heart disease, by raising the good HDL cholesterol.

And last but not least, is your lifetime **Fit-Step® Walking Program.** Walking not only provides cardiovascular fitness, but as we have seen it also raises the HDL (good cholesterol-submarine) level in our blood. HDL seems to protect our coronary arteries from accumulating too much cholesterol.

THE GOOD, THE BAD AND THE UGLY

Trans-fatty acids, commonly called *trans-fats,* are found in cooking oil, margarine, shortening and processed foods. They are formed when hydrogen atoms are added to oils containing mono or polyunsaturated fats. The hydrogenation process converts liquid oils into a more solid form. Several studies have shown that trans-fats can raise the LDL cholesterol by nearly as much, if not more, as those foods that are high in saturated fats. You should avoid deep fried foods, french fries, doughnuts, stick margarines and other products which are labeled partially hydrogenated oils, which is another term for trans-fats. You should cook with olive oil and use soft margarines sparingly that do not have trans-fats on the label which would be listed as partially hydrogenated oil. Polyunsaturated fats are the *good fats*. Monosaturated fats are the *better fats*. Saturated fats are the *bad fats*. And trans-fats are the sneaky, *ugly fats*.

THE SEVEN COUNTRIES STUDY

One of the most striking studies on the relationship of *serum cholesterol* to development of *coronary heart disease* is illustrated in *The Seven Countries Study*. This study was a collaborative international study of more than *12,000 women and men, ages 40 to 59 years of age*. Its purpose was to relate the characteristics of these populations to the subsequent development of coronary heart disease. Total communities were involved in the following countries: Greece, Yugoslavia, Italy, Japan, Finland, The Netherlands and the United States.

Dietary differences studied in The Seven Countries Study revealed that people in Japan and the Mediterranean countries consumed a diet containing *10 percent or less* calories daily from saturated fat, whereas the diet in the United States, Finland and The Netherlands contained *15 to 22 percent saturated fat*. In the countries that consumed a diet containing 10 percent or less calories from saturated fat, their dietary consumption of complex carbohydrates and vegetable protein from grains, vegetables, legumes and fruits was significantly higher than in the countries which had a higher intake of saturated fat. The blood cholesterol of people in the *Mediterranean countries and Japan was 200 mg.* or less, whereas in the *United States, Finland and The Netherlands*, whose intake of saturated fats was approximately 20 percent of calories, the blood cholesterol levels ranged from *230 to 265 mg*.

The *cholesterol blood levels* in the seven countries studied were directly correlated with the incidence of *coronary heart disease*.

Japan, which had the lowest incidence of coronary heart disease in this study, had the lowest blood cholesterol level of about 160 mg. *Finland,* on the other hand, had the highest rate of coronary heart disease and had the highest serum cholesterol level, approximately 260 mg. The ten year mortality from coronary heart disease was lowest in *Japan* and the three *Mediterranean countries* (Yugoslavia, Greece and Italy). The highest rates were found in the *United States, Finland and The Netherlands.*

There can be little doubt from this intensive, exhaustive study that the level of serum cholesterol, which is directly related to the intake of *saturated fat and dietary cholesterol* is a prime risk factor in the development of *coronary heart disease.* <u>Don't let any- one try to fool you by stating that low carbohydrate, high-fat diets are good for you.</u> It's plain nonsense! And you have seven countries around the world to prove that a high fat diet is dangerous to your health.

20 LOW FAT TIPS

1. When shopping, go to the market after you've eaten, so you won't buy impulse high fat snack foods. Buy only items on a prepared list that you make before marketing. Don't deviate from this list with snack foods, which you might have a ten- dency to buy, if you had not eaten prior to marketing.

2. When shopping for packaged or canned goods, make sure the item of food you are purchasing has no more than 1.5 - 2.0 grams of total fat. If it is higher, look for another brand. Always look for non-fat or low-fat products; however, remember to look at the label, and don't depend on a label that says low-fat food. Many so-called low-fat items are fairly high in total fat content; for example 2% milk has 5 grams of fat, or 98% fat free yogurt can have 3.5 to 4 grams of total fat. Always choose foods that are less than 2.0 grams of total fat. Also watch out for labels that say "cholesterol-free." These foods may have 0 grams of cholesterol; however, they may contain many grams of total fat.

3. Don't use foods as a stress reliever. Women have a tendency to seek out high-fat, high-sugar foods when under stress. Substitute music, exercise, meditation or a warm bath for food cravings.

4. Make your meals attractive with colorful foods, garnishes and greens, carrots, tomatoes, broccoli, spinach, peppers, yams, celery, parsley, etc. in order to make them more appealing and vary your menu plans daily to avoid boredom. Remember that the more colorful the foods are, the more phyto-nutrients they contain.

5. Foods should be kept out of sight between meals in your refrigerator or pantry.

6. Women who skip breakfast usually wind up with a high fat, high-sugar snack (example doughnut and coffee mid-morning.) A high fiber, low-fat cereal with fruit and skim milk will hold you comfortably until lunchtime.

7. Fresh vegetables and fruits are better choices than canned fruits and vegetables, which can be loaded with salt or sugar.

8. Soups and stews can be loaded with hidden fats. Refrigerate them overnight after preparing, and skim off the layer of fat that is lying on the surface of the stew or soup. You'll be removing more than $3/4$ of the fat contained in these products. Choose soups loaded with vegetables and beans, and avoid any soups that are cream-based.

9. Drink at least six 8 oz. glasses of water daily. Avoid drinking a lot of artificially sweetened drinks as they can increase your appetite, due to the hypoglycemic effect (it lowers your blood sugar).

10. Cream, whole milk, or powdered creamers should be avoided in coffee or tea. Substitute skim milk. Non-fat dairy creams are O.K.

11. Low fat, non-fat, or part skim-milk cheeses should be substituted for all other cheese. Make sure, however, that you check the total fat content per serving size.

12. Baked potato is an excellent food for meals or snacks (high fiber, low fat), compared to french fries, which are saturated with up to 15 grams of fat per serving. However, if you have a craving for french fries, you can prepare low-fat french fries by slicing potatoes, spraying with non-fat vegetable spray, and baking for 20-30 minutes in an oven at approximately 300 degrees, or microwaving for 3 to 5 minutes. Keep your portion size small.

13. Use a rack to roast meat, poultry or fish. The fat drips off during cooking. Baste with broth or vegetable juice to preserve moisture. Never use butter, margarine, shortening, or gravy mixes. Defatted chicken broth is a good alternative.

14. Trim all visible skin and fat from poultry and meat before cooking.

15. Fresh or canned beans of any variety are excellent sources of fiber and vitamins. Their low fat content makes them excellent companions to any meal. Make sure they are not prepared with meat (example: baked beans with bacon.) Avoid high fat refried beans; however, several companies now have non-fat refried beans available.

16. Fruits and vegetable skins are excellent sources of fiber, as well as the seeds, (berries, tomatoes, cucumbers, and pumpkins.)

17. Avoid sugar, sodas, teas, and fruit drinks. Use fresh orange juice,

grapefruit juice, tomato juice (low sodium), and non-caffeinated teas, coffee and sodas for snack drinks. Make plain old water (tap or bottled) as your drink of choice. Remember to drink at least six 8 oz. glasses of water daily.

18. Skim milk, which has no fat, has all of the calcium, vitamins and minerals that are present in 1%, 2%, or whole milk, and it tastes just as good.

19. Non-fat yogurt is an excellent source of calcium and its lactobacillus, and other cultures are friendly bacteria for your colon.

20. Breads that are high in fiber, low in fat are the following: whole grain, bran-enriched, cracked wheat, whole-wheat pita, rye, pumpernickel and those labeled high fiber breads. High fat, low fiber breads are French, Italian, white, garlic bread, rolls and bagels: Stay away from them. Remember to check the ingredients label. If the first ingredient doesn't say "whole," then it is not a whole-grain, high fiber bread.

MORE LOW FAT TIPS

1. A tasty non-fat dessert is angel food cake with fresh fruit and non-fat whipped cream. (A slice of cheese or chocolate cake has up to 14 grams of fat). The angel food cake as described above has less than 1.5 grams.

2. Sherbet, sorbet, frozen fruit bars and non-fat frozen yogurts are excellent substitutes for your ice cream sweet tooth.

3. Salad dressings and mayonnaise are no-no's in the Diet Step® 20/20 plan. Substitute non-fat dressings or non-fat mayonnaise. If not available, either use no dressing, or just dip your fork gently into the dressing on the side every 2-3 bites of salad, and you'll get the taste without the added fat calories.

4. Non-fat popcorn is an excellent low-fat, high fiber snack. Don't add butter or salt. Use hot air popper or microwave non-fat varieties.

5. When eating out, choose low-fat foods without sauces, like broiled fish or chicken with a large tossed salad. Avoid alcohols, since they can increase your appetite, and add extra calories. Incidentally, one gram of alcohol contains 9 calories, higher than a gram of fat, carbohydrate, or protein. If you definitely like a drink with dinner, a wine spritzer is a good substitute, which is relatively low in total calorie value. However, 4 oz. of red wine or a light beer is permitted on the Diet-Step® Plan every other night.

6. At parties, weddings, etc., concentrate on the fresh vegetables without the dips, and fresh fruits. Avoid those fat-laden little appetizers with toothpicks in them. They're warning red flags to stay away!

7. When traveling by air, order ahead for a low-fat meal when making reservations. They're available! Otherwise, if it is a short flight, have a low-fat snack prior to boarding.

8. Non-stick pans use less fat than cast iron, copper or aluminum pans. Use non-stick vegetable sprays as the first choice; otherwise, a small amount of olive oil (1 tsp.) or canola oil can be used for cooking.

9. Grilled or broiled foods, which include vegetables, fish, poultry and lean meats, are tasty low-fat dishes. The fat drips away as the foods are cooked. A light dusting of olive oil is all that is necessary, and many companies now make olive oil sprays which use considerably less fat than the tablespoon method.

10. Steamed vegetables, with or without herbs, can be cooked in a basket over boiling water. Steaming retains the flavor, color and nutrients of the vegetable.

11. Poaching fish in water at a simmer (just below the boiling point of water) preserves the taste and texture of the fish. Any condiments can be added to the liquid to enhance the flavor, such as garlic or herbs.

12. Stir-frying in a pan or wok is a fast way to make tasty vegetables, chicken, meats or fish. Add very small amounts of olive or peanut oil and seasonings followed by either defatted chicken broth or low-sodium soy sauce.

13. Sautéing: Use non-stick, non-fat vegetable sprays or a small amount of wine or defatted broth. Vegetables, fish, poultry or meats are mixed together in a pan. Then add herbs, such as thyme, basil, sage, or dill, for added taste.

14. Microwaving food uses the foods' own moisture to cook. It's quick and easy, and you don't have to add any fat when microwaving. Almost all foods are microwaveable.

15. Peeling a potato (white or sweet potato) before cooking or eating removes more than 25% of its nutrients and 35-40% of its fiber.

16. If you put salt on poultry, fish or meat before cooking, the food loses a good portion of its vitamin and mineral content during the cooking process. This is because the added salt causes the food to be drained of its nutrients during the cooking process, which end up in the cooking broth.

17. Don't be afraid to send back your meal in a restaurant if they didn't follow your instructions for your order. For example, if you asked for steamed vegetables, baked potato, and broiled fish without butter, that's the way it should arrive on your plate.

18. Pasta: Spaghetti or linguini are lower in fat than wider pastas that are often made with eggs. Try to order (restaurant) or buy whole grain pasta or spinach noodles for their high-fiber content. Stick to tomato or marinara sauces (Some, however, have much too much oil, and you can have the waiter drain the oil from the pasta and bring back your dish) or seafood--based sauces without cream are also good substitutes.

19. Pizza can be ordered without cheese (tomato pie) and then add on a variety of fresh vegetables. If you want cheese, sprinkle on a little Parmesan cheese.

20. Chinese restaurants: Stir-fry foods are better than deep-fried. Choose dishes with grains and vegetables. Order brown rice instead of white rice for the extra fiber content (not fried rice, which also comes out brown in color but is low in fiber). Ask to have your food prepared without soy sauce or MSG. Choose vegetable wonton soup or any vegetable-based soup rather than meat-based soups.

21. Mexican foods are great, if you can stay away from the deep-fried tortilla chips and order oven-baked chips with salsa instead. Skip the sour cream and guacamole (avocado) both of which are high in fat. Soft corn tortillas (tostadas or enchiladas) with chicken, tomato sauce and onions are good low-fat choices. Burritos or fajitas without sour cream or guacamole are excellent choices with lettuce, tomato and onion, and can be considered low-fat dishes. Avoid regular refried beans, deep-fried chimichangas, beef taco salad and deep-fried tortilla chips.

22. Choose whole wheat or oat bran English muffins, whole wheat rolls or bread, whole wheat or oat bran bagels or raisin bread instead of sweet rolls, doughnuts, cakes and white bread. Tip: always scoop-out inside of rolls or bagels.

23. Fat-free snacks: dried or fresh fruits, raisins, peaches, apples,

plums, apricots, bananas or baby carrots and celery stalks.

24. Hard pretzels (non-fat) and soft pretzels (non-fat). For example, Superpretzel®, rice cakes (flavored) or hot-air popped corn are excellent low-fat snacks.

25. Spreads for breads: jelly, honey, fruit preserves and all fruit jams instead of margarine or butter.

26. Baked potatoes or corn chips (non-fat) in place of french fries or potato chips.

FAT IS WHERE IT'S AT

At a recent American Heart Association meeting, a study showed that men and women store fat in different places: men are more likely to store fat in their abdomens, whereas women store fat more easily in their buttocks and thighs, because nature gave women more fat cells there. What's the significance of these findings? Extra abdominal fat increases the risk of stroke, high blood pressure, diabetes and high cholesterol levels. The extra fat stored by women in the thighs and buttocks appear to be a harmless place to store fat according to this study; however, no woman wants to have fat thighs and buttocks. The good news is that women who walk seem to lose weight more easily in those trouble spots, the thighs and buttocks, making these areas firm and trim. So no matter whether the fat's in your belly or in your buttocks, *walking women stay slim and trim.*

YO-YO DIETS--NO-NO!

The Framingham Heart Study, which has followed more than 5,000 people for almost 40 years, recently indicated a health hazard for chronic dieters. People who lost 10% of their body weight had an almost 20% reduction in the incidence of heart disease. So what's the problem? These same dieters who gained back the 10% of their body weight, *raised their heart disease risk by almost* 30%. So if you weigh 160 lbs. and lost 10% or 16 lbs., you decreased your heart disease risk by 20%. But if you gained back that 16 lbs., you increased your risk of heart attack by 30%, an overall net gain of 10% and you still weigh the same 160 lbs. *Sounds scary to me, folks!* How many times have you heard the old saying that "I've lost enough weight over the years to equal two or three whole persons and I've gained every bit of it back." *Yo-yo dieting or weight-cycling* makes it harder to permanently lose weight and is much more dangerous to your health.

Experts in the fields of physiology, biochemistry, psychology, nutrition and medicine have come up with the following startling findings about yo-yo dieting:

1. The weight-loss/weight-gain cycle *actually increases your desire for fatty foods.* Animal research studies at Yale University showed that rats who had lost weight rapidly on low-calorie diets, always chose more fat in their diets when given a choice between fat, protein, and carbohydrates. These rats always put on more weight than when they started and in a much shorter time than it had taken them to lose the weight.

2. Yo-yo dieters *increase the percentage of body fat* to lean body tissue with repeated bouts of weight gain and weight loss. Women who lose weight rapidly on a low carbohydrate-high protein diet can lose a significant amount of muscle tissue. If the weight is regained again, they usually regain more fat and less muscle because it is easier for the body to gain fat than it is to rebuild muscle tissue.

3. *Body fat gets redistributed in the abdomen* from the thighs, buttocks and hips after weight cycling. Medical research has definitely shown that fat deposits above the waist increases the risk of heart disease and diabetes, not to mention an unsightly paunch.

4. When you lose weight by cutting calories, your *basal metabolic rate (BMR)* goes down, because it is the body's defense mechanism against starvation. The body can't tell the difference between starvation and low calorie dieting; consequently, your body is trying to conserve energy by burning fewer calories. This is the reason it becomes harder to lose weight after a week or two, even though you are eating exactly the same amount of calories as you did when you first started your diet. This slow-down in the basal metabolic rate (BMR) persists even after the diet is over and accounts for the rapid-rebound, excessive weight gain that always happens to the dieter when she goes off her diet. This slow-down in metabolic rate can occur even after a single attempt at dieting. However, the repeated effects of weight-cycling diets can affect the basal metabolic rate (BMR) much more, making additional weight-loss almost impossible and rebound weight gain almost inevitable. The yo-yo dieter is often heard to say -- "I'm heavier now than I was before I started this damn diet."

5. An enzyme called *lipoprotein lipase (LPL)* becomes more active when you cut calories. This enzyme controls the amount of fat that is stored in your body's fat cells. Dieting, therefore, makes the body more efficient at storing fat, which is exactly the opposite of what a dieter wants. As you reduce your calorie intake, the enzyme LPL starts to activate the fat-storing process. This is another defense mechanism that the body uses to prevent starvation. Remember, the enzyme LPL doesn't know that you are dieting; it thinks that you are starving to death.

6. Women dieters who've lost a substantial amount of weight were compared to women of normal weight. After they lost weight, the previously obese women needed surprisingly fewer calories to maintain their weight than the normal-weight women. In this study, obese women who lost weight needed only 2000 calories a day to maintain their weight (125 lbs.) compared to 2300 calories

per day to maintain the exact same weight (125 lbs.) by normal-weight people. Who said dieting was fair?

7. Chronic female dieters who exhibited repeated cycles of weight gain and weight loss showed an increased risk of sudden death from heart attacks, according to a recent medical report. This study followed 1500 women over a period of 25 years who had engaged in cyclic-dieting.

So what's the answer? We know that losing weight lowers blood pressure, reduces the risk of heart disease, lowers blood cholesterol and triglycerides and increases the HDL ("good" cholesterol). The answer is that dieting alone is not the best way to lose and maintain weight. The following is a list of the reasons why *walking, combined with the Diet-Step® Diet Plan is the only safe and effective method* to lose and maintain normal body weight:

1. Exercise, particularly walking, is the real answer to preventing the weight loss/weight-gain cycle from occurring. Walking makes it less likely you'll gain the weight back again because you lose more fat and less muscle tissue with exercise. Also, walking prevents the slow-down in basal metabolic rate that always occurs with a yo-yo diet. Actually walking slightly increases the BMR, which helps to burn calories at a faster rate. Walking also reduces the production of the enzyme lipoprotein lipase (LPL), which in turn decreases the amount of fat stored in the fat cells.

2. Walking also regulates the brain's *appetite* controller, the appestat. The more you walk, the more you decrease the appestat's hunger mechanism. Inactivity, on the other hand, stimulates the appetite control mechanism to make you hungry.

3. Walking, by increasing the aerobic metabolism of the body, redirects the stomach's blood supply to the exercising muscles, which in turn decreases your appetite.

4. And finally, walking encourages the body to burn fat rather than carbohydrates. This enables the body's blood sugar to stay at a relatively constant normal level. When the brain's blood sugar is normal we are not hungry. Both strenuous exercise and low-calorie dieting, however, burn carbohydrates rather than fats, causing a sharp drop in the blood sugar. When the brain's blood sugar drops as it does in dieting or strenuous exercises, then we feel hungry in order to counteract this low blood sugar. The high fiber content of the Diet-Step® diet also controls the body's appetite center, making over-eating high-fat calories next to impossible.

By combining the <u>Diet-Step®: 20 Grams Fat/20 Grams Fiber Diet</u> with the <u>Fit-Step® 20 minute walking plan,</u> you have the most effective method of losing and maintaining your weight without the dangers of yo-yo dieting.

SMALL FREQUENT MEALS BURN FAT FASTER

After a meal, the pancreas (an endocrine gland located behind your stomach) produces a hormone called insulin, which is released into the bloodstream. A meal that is high in fat or sugar causes the pancreas to release a lot more insulin than does a meal which is high in complex carbohydrates. Likewise, a larger meal causes more insulin to be released than a smaller meal. One of insulin's functions is to regulate the level of sugar in the blood by burning carbohydrates and conserving stores of body fat. In other words, high levels of insulin prevent the release of fat from the body's fat cells into the blood, where it could be burned as fuel for energy. As you can see, then, this is not a good thing, because the fat stays in the fat cells and you stay fat while you're trying to diet. Also, high levels of insulin promote the absorption of dietary fat into the body's fat cells. In other words, the higher the level of insulin, the more fat that is absorbed into your fat cells and the less fat that can get out of the cells.

More frequent, smaller meals, on the other hand, tend to keep the pancreas from producing excess amounts of insulin. This results in more dietary fat being burned as fuel, which results in less fat being stored in the fat cells. Also, less insulin encourages the breakdown of fat already in your fat cells to be released into the blood to be used as an additional fuel for energy. In other words, small, frequent complex-carbohydrate meals as on the Diet--Step® 20/20 Plan produce steady, lower levels of insulin being released into the bloodstream than does eating larger, high-fat, high sugar meals. Therefore, small, frequent complex carbohydrate meals result in more fat being burned as a fuel and less fat being stored as fat deposits. As an added benefit of eating small, frequent complex carbohydrate meals, you actually produce a decrease in your appetite. This is due to the fact that as you burn more fat, you are actually using up calories, instead of storing calories.

DANGEROUS DIETING

The low carbohydrate craze, which is essentially a high-fat diet, has been seen recently in a variety of different diet books all proposing the same low carbohydrate diet. Any diet that restricts carbohydrates will definitely cause weight loss in the first few days of the diet. However, the weight loss is not from fat loss. Most all of the weight that is lost in the early period of the diet is lean tissue, water and essential minerals. All of these elements are vitally important to the body, and if the body were to continue to lose lean tissue at a rapid rate, then disease, disability and death would occur within a month's time.

In order to prevent this dangerous condition from occurring, the body shifts into an abnormal metabolic state called ketosis. In ketosis, fatty acids are broken down to form ketones and acetones, which the body can then use as fuel. Unfortunately, this results in the loss of sodium and potassium from the body, which are vital minerals essential for health. Even levels of thyroid hormone decrease and your metabolism slows down to conserve energy, which in turn, slows the process of weight loss. During this process of ketosis, the blood cholesterol goes up, which in itself, is a dangerous condition. While the body is breaking down fat to form ketones for energy, it must consume some of its lean tissue to meet the energy needs of the brain and nervous system. Since the brain and nervous system use approximately 2/3 of the glucose present in the body, ketones cannot replace glucose for many of the brain's functions. This, in turn, can affect the brain adversely, since lean tissue must be broken down to form amino acids, which can then be converted to glucose. If this is not done in a timely fashion, then the brain's blood supply of glucose is limited, resulting in temporary and/or permanent neurological damage.

Since this diet is primarily animal protein, you are shorting yourself on vitamins, minerals, antioxidants, phyto-chemicals, essential fatty acids and fiber. These important nutrients, which are primarily found in plant foods (vegetables, grains and fruits), have been proven to protect and prevent heart disease, cancer, strokes and a variety of other degenerative diseases. The more animal fat that you consume with this diet, the more you increase your risk of cardiovascular and cerebrovascular disease, since the blood lipids, in particular cholesterol and lipoproteins, become elevated. As you can see, this is a dangerous way to diet and is not a healthy type of diet to remain on for any period of time. In addition, once this diet is stopped, rapid weight gain resumes, since the body has been depleted of water and nutrients. The appestat (hunger center) in the brain increases and you usually begin to consume massive quantities of carbohydrates to alleviate the adverse effects of this diet.

The Diet-Step® Plan, which includes 20 grams of fat and 20 grams of fiber, is a safe, effective diet plan in which you can lose weight, maintain your weight easily, feel healthy, more energetic and live a longer life. In addition, the weight loss in this diet plan is permanent, not temporary, and does not cause any abnormal body aberrations which can affect your metabolism or your health. Bon Appetit!

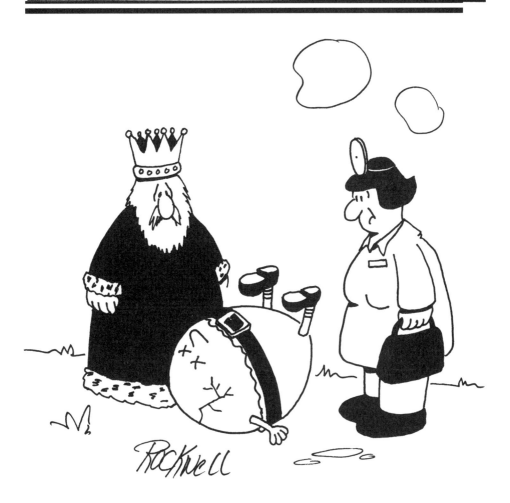

"I THINK IT WAS THE FALL THAT KILLED HIM. ALTHOUGH, HE DID HAVE A VERY HIGH CHOLESTEROL."

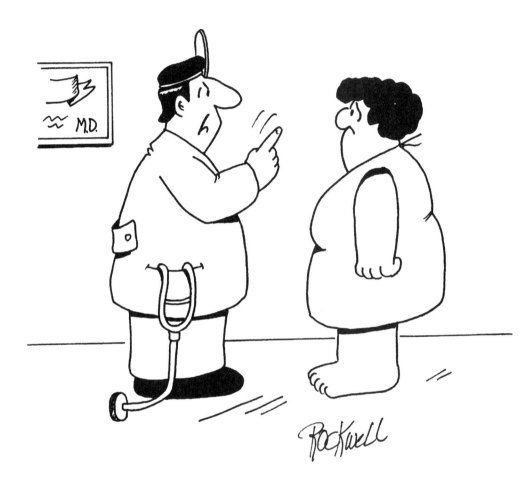

"WHAT DO YOU MEAN, I OUGHT TO BE ON A DIET TOO? I'M THE DOCTOR."

CHAPTER 5

DIET FACTS AND FALLACIES
****

1. **Calories don't count. False!** This is the first of the many falla-cies that people use in the weight-loss business. On the con-trary, calories do count in a weight-gain, weight-loss program. In order to gain or lose a pound of fat you must eat or not eat *3,500* more calories than you use up. However, in the Diet-Step®: 20/Grams Fat/20 Grams Fiber Diet, there is no need to count calories, since they're automatically factored into the Diet-Step®: 20/Grams Fat/20 Grams Fiber quick weight loss plan.

2. **A crash diet** is an excellent way to begin a weight-loss pro-gram. **False!** This is probably the worst way to begin a diet pro-gram since most crash diets, which are usually low in carbohy-drates, produce rapid fluid loss. This fluid loss has nothing to do with the amount of liquid that we drink, and it is only reflect-ing a change in the body's ability to hold fluid. The fallacy is that fat is not coming off in this type of program, and, in fact, protein can be lost during a crash diet, which may be harmful to the kidneys. When these diets are abandoned, weight is gained rapidly, usually in the form of fat, and the dieter may wind up with more fat than when she started.

3. **Exercise is unimportant** in weight reduction and control. **False!** Nothing can be further from the truth. Regular physical exercise and activity is the key point in a long-term weight maintenance program. Exercise not only burns calories, but has an appetite-regulating effect on the brain's appetite-control mechanism. Exercise also favorably affects the metabolism by lowering blood pressure, blood cholesterol, blood sugar and in general, contributing to good health.

4. **Eating more in the morning** will put on less weight than eating food in the evening. **False!** The body does not distinguish between time of day and calories consumed. It's the total amount of calories that you consume daily that determines your weight.

5. **Certain foods can burn up calories,** such as grapefruit. **False!** This is entirely erroneous. The digestion of food does consume some energy from the process of digestion, but there is no food that expends enough energy during digestion to promote weight loss.

6. **It is better to smoke than be fat. False!** The initial weight gained from decreasing or stopping smoking can always be lost by a diet and exercise program; however, the permanent lung, heart and artery damage done by smoking can never be undone.

7. **Toasting bread reduces its calorie count. False!** Toasting only changes the bread's texture and taste but does not burn away calories.

8. **It does not make any difference whether you eat slowly or quickly as far as appetite or weight gain are concerned. False!** Eating a meal slowly and chewing the food thoroughly gives the body's metabolism a chance to regulate and reduce its appetite-regulating center in the brain. This subsequently can reduce the appetite and make you more satisfied with less food. Eating rapidly does not cause overweight; however, since many overweight people tend to eat rapidly and do not give the appetite suppressing mechanism time to work, they eat more.

9. **Since meat** is **high in protein, it does not cause weight gain. False!** Protein, no matter what the source, contains 4 calories per gram. Carbohydrate also contains four calories per gram. Fat, however, contains nine calories per gram, more than twice as many calories as a gram of protein or carbohydrate. Since any excessive calories above the body's basic metabolic

requirements results in an increased storage of fat, eating meat not only can cause weight gain but can cause a greater proportion of fat being deposited in the body because of its high fat content. Therefore, meat not only gives four calories per gram for its protein content, but it also gives nine calories per gram for its fat content. Therefore, the greater the percentage of fat in the meat, the higher the caloric value.

10. **Since protein is the most important nutritional requirement of the body, high protein diets are the most beneficial and the healthiest. False!** Protein is a very important part of the body and is necessary in the diet for providing the amino acids (building blocks) for cellular activity, tissue repair and general maintenance of the body. However, protein is not the only essential requirement of our bodies. Carbohydrates, fats, vitamins, minerals, essential fatty acids and calories are necessary to provide energy and the basic ingredients to work the body's physiological and biochemical machinery properly. High protein diets are also high in total fat and saturated fats, which are deadly for your arteries.

11. **As long as you take a vitamin supplement every day, it doesn't matter what foods you eat or drink. False!** Vitamin supplements will not provide all the daily requirements of protein, carbohydrates, minerals, amino acids and essential fatty acids that the body needs. This is a widespread misconception about nutrition and dieting. Many complications have been noted by people on very low calorie diets combined with protein-vitamin supplements, because of the inability of the body's metabolism, particularly the kidneys and liver, to adjust to this type of diet.

12. **If I skip breakfast and lunch and just eat a large supper, I will lose weight. False!** No matter when the calories are consumed in a given 24-hour period the total end result is the same. The basic formula is: calories consumed vs. calories expended; whether you eat 400 calories three times a day or 1,200 calories

at one meal, the body does not know the difference. In addition, skipping meals is not a healthful way to embark on a diet program, since the appetite becomes over-stimulated late in the day and you not only eat a large dinner but you also eat continuous snacks throughout the evening.

13. **If I eat or snack at bedtime, the food will not be digested properly and I will gain weight. False!** Again, the same principle exists as to the total calories consumed in any 24-hour period vs. the total calories expended. This is the basic formula needed for either weight gain, weight loss, or weight maintenance. Eating at bedtime will not put any more weight on than eating at any other time of day or night. Some people, however, may develop indigestion when they eat immediately before bedtime.

14. **Liver and red meat are essential in the diet because of their high content of iron. False!** While liver and red meat are excellent sources of iron as well as other nutrients, including protein, vitamin A, niacin, and riboflavin, they also have a high content of saturated fats and are not a necessary part of any dietary program. There are many other foods, including green leafy vegetables, chicken, turkey and fish, which have adequate quantities of iron without the high saturated fat content.

A BAKER'S DOZEN GREAT DIET TIPS

1. **Eat more slowly with each meal.** This involves taking smaller, less frequent bites and chewing each mouthful for a longer period of time. Pause between each section of the meal.

2. If you are still hungry when you are finished your first portion, **wait at least fifteen minutes** to see whether or not you really want another portion. In most cases your appestat (the brain appetite control mechanism) will be more than satisfied at the end of that period of time and you will not need a second helping.

3. Also restrict your meals to one, or perhaps two, locations in your home for eating. If you have no regular place to eat, then you will find that you are eating in every room; however, when food is restricted to **one main dining area,** there will be less tendency to snack during the day.

4. Make sure you leave **the table as soon as** you are finished eating and spend less **time in the kitchen** or areas that have a tendency to remind one of eating.

5. Make sure that you do not place **serving dishes** on the table during a meal for there will be more of a tendency to take second and third helpings. Be sure that you **do not leave food out** where you can repeatedly see it during the day.

6. Never go to the market on an empty stomach; you will buy snack foods (carbohydrate cravings). Also make it a point not to eat while watching **television** or **reading** since you will eat more while not concentrating on your meal.

7. Remember not to start a weight reduction program just prior to the **holiday season** or before **vacation time** since these are the most unsuccessful times to begin this type of project.

8. **Fried foods** should be avoided, since, even though you drain excess fat away, the fried foods still retain a large percentage of fat, which adds to the calories. **Boiling, broiling, baking, or steaming** are the best techniques for preparing foods.

9. **Fat on poultry and meat:** Always trim away visible fat from meat and fowl before cooking and remove visible fat at the table when eating. The skin of the chicken contains 25 percent of the fat content of the chicken and will add tremendously to the calories. Canned fishes, such as tuna and salmon, should be packed in water or the oils drained away.

10. **Hot foods** such as soups, and foods that require a lot of **chewing** will leave you with a greater feeling of satisfaction because they take a longer time to swallow and absorb. Make sure you **leave the table** as soon as you finish eating.

11. Eat salad **greens** and **vegetables** before the main course since these will take the edge off your hunger for higher calorie meat, poultry and fish portions. The best salad dressing is none. Salad dressings are high in fats and calories. Use calorie-free herbs spices, lemon, vinegar, or occasionally a small amount (one tsp.) non-fat, low-calorie dressing. **Restaurant tip:** Dip your fork in a side cup of salad dressing every 3-4 mouthfuls of salad and you'll enjoy the taste without the extra calories.

12. **Teflon coated pans** and the new non-fat **edible spray-on coatings,** which are made of vegetable oil, will help reduce the amount of caloric fat that you consume. Although **margarine** is lower in saturated fats than butter, it is still 100 percent fat and has almost as many calories as butter, not to mention the bad fats (trans-fats).

13. **Alcohol:** Alcohol is one of the most serious hazards in any diet program, whether it is dining out or at home. The additional calories which are consumed in the American diet from alcohol have a tendency to cause and maintain overweight problems. Alcohol has more calories (seven calories per gram) than most foods on a weight basis. Try to substitute club soda with a twist of lemon or mineral water for drinks. However, you're allowed 4 oz. red wine or 12 oz. light beer 3 days per week on the Diet-Step® plan.

WHY DO WE GET FOOD CRAVINGS?

Food cravings may have a **physiological** as well as an **emotional** component, according to many researchers. Those eating binges or cravings for ice cream, pizza, and hoagies may not necessarily begin in the stomach.

CARBOHYDRATE CRAVINGS for sweets, cakes, pretzels, potato chips and crackers may be caused *by low blood sugar.* This condition can occur when you have not eaten for several hours or because of emotional frustration and has been noted to be present prior to the menstrual period because of hormonal fluctuations. Complex carbohydrates like fruits, vegetables and whole-grain cereal grains can reduce the craving for refined carbohydrates. High protein-non-fat milk and low-fat (skim milk) cheese can also cut this craving.

SALT CRAVINGS such as pickles, potato chips, and olives can result from a *salt depletion* caused by excessive perspiration, or a *stress condition* which results in the stimulation of the adrenal glands. Salt cravings can be reduced by substituting lemon juice and herbs and adding fresh fruit (orange, grapefruit, banana, cantaloupe, tomatoes or strawberries) to the diet which has a *high vitamin-C content,* which can reduce the craving for salt.

CAFFEINE is present in coffee, tea, cola drinks, cocoa and chocolate which contains theobromine (a caffeine-type substance). Many people are actually *addicted* both physiologically and metabolically to caffeine and will suffer emotional *withdrawal symptoms,* which include headache, fatigue, nausea, irritability and even a craving for sugar. To reduce this addiction you have to gradually reduce the caffeine in your diet by substituting *non-caffeine* drinks such as decaffeinated coffee, herbal teas, clear diet sodas other than colas, and mineral water or club soda.

THOSE SNEAKY, HIDDEN FATS KEEP GETTING IN OUR FOOD

The typical American diet is considerably higher in fat content than nearly any other country in the world. There is little doubt that this increased fat intake in our diet is responsible for such diseases as heart disease, obesity, cancers of the colon, breast and prostate. *Fat* is the most concentrated source of calories since a gram of dietary fat supplies your body with *nine calories*. This compares to only four calories per gram of protein or carbohydrate. Alcohol has seven calories per gram, slightly less than fat, but more than carbohydrate or protein. Since fat has this concentrated source of calories, it is the *most fattening type of food* that we consume and it stands to reason that cutting down on the fat intake is one of the best ways to cut down on the total amount of calories and maintain normal body weight.

Fat accounted for approximately 30 percent of our calories in the early 1900's, whereas today, the fat content of our diet has more than *40 percent* of our calories coming from fat. In order to meet the basic nutritional requirements, we need only eat one tablespoon of *polyunsaturated oil* each day, which supplies the essential fatty acid called *linoleic acid.* This essential fatty acid helps you absorb fat-soluble vitamins. Americans, however, eat six to eight times this amount of fat, and fat can be considered to be the major source of nutritionally empty calories for most Americans.

Americans have become more conscious of fat consumption in the past ten years; however, only about a third of the fat we eat is *visible* fat, such as hard fat on meat, fats and oils used in cooking, and oil-based salad dressings. Most of the fat in our diet, unfortunately, is hidden fat and not as readily noticeable as the marbled fat on meat. *Hidden fat,* unfortunately, is a major part of hard cheeses, cream cheese, deep- fried foods, creamed soups, ice cream, chocolate, nuts and seeds. Hidden fat is also a major ingredient of processed, prepared foods such as baked goods (pies, cakes and cookies), processed meats (bologna, hot dogs, etc.), coffee creamers, whipped toppings, snack foods and instant meals. Many health food products which are purchased as substitutes for saturated fats have in themselves high fat content. Nuts and seeds, sesame paste, granola, quiches and avocados may contain more than half the calories as fat calories.

REDUCING FAT IN YOUR DIET

When shopping in the market, it is often difficult to tell how much fat is contained in the processed foods. Always check the label for the ingredients and remember that the *ingredients are listed in order of their weight.* Therefore, if fat or oil is listed as one of the first two ingredients, then the product is likely to be high in fat, especially if it precedes the flour content, for example, in baked goods. The *Nutritional Facts* label will tell you how much total fat and saturated fat is in each serving and what the serving size is. Trans-fats (bad fats) aren't listed since there is no current requirement to label trans-fatty acids in food products. Trans-fat is produced when unsaturated fat is hydrogenated, turning it into a solid. Next, check the *Ingredients* label. If hydrogenated or partially hydrogenated fat is listed, then a pretty good estimate is to consider that in most hydrogenated food products, the trans-fat content probably equals the saturated fat on the label. So, if 2 grams of saturated fat is listed on the label, you can double that amount making it 4 grams per serving.

FATS

Whipped margarine and butter contain less fat per serving than regular margarine or butter because air or water replaces some of the fat in these products. A tablespoon of mayonnaise or oil may have as many fat calories as a teaspoon of hard fat; however, the softer, more liquid fats are less saturated. It is far better to choose the newer soft spreads that are labeled oil-free, which contain no trans-fats.

DAIRY PRODUCTS

Low fat, one percent milk or skim milk is preferable to any other milk product. Low fat yogurt, cottage cheese and ricotta cheese are preferable to other diary products. Parmesan and mozzarella cheese made from skim milk have less fat than hard cheeses. Sour cream and sweet cream both are high in fat content and should be avoided. Use skim milk if you are preparing puddings or custards from a packaged mix. Ice milk and frozen yogurt have less fat than ice cream and milkshakes. Soft ice cream, such as frozen custard may contain as much fat as the hard varieties. Buttermilk contains little or no butterfat and can be used in baked goods to add taste and richness.

SALADS

Salads are fine for the low fat diet, provided they are made without dressings; use herbs and spices. Occasionally adding lemon juice with the spices will be satisfactory. There are also low calorie salad dressings which can be used; however, they too have a considerable fat content. The newer non-fat salad dressings are preferable. Also, wine-vinegar is a tasty salad dressing when mixed with 1/2 tsp. olive oil.

SOUPS

Clear consommé broth and clear soup made with noodles, beans, rice or vegetables are preferable to creamed soups or heavy stock soups.

MEATS

Heavily marbled prime cuts of meats and processed meats are the highest in fat content. Sirloin tip, london broil and flank steak are leaner than the heavily marbled beef. Veal and leg of lamb are also lean. Always buy lean hamburger. Never fry meats, always broil or grill. Avoid gravies and cream sauces. Make gravy at home after skimming off the fat.

FISH

Tuna and salmon, surprisingly, are among the fattier fishes. However, they contain the heart-protective 3-omega fatty acids that are good for you. Sardines in oil and many forms of smoked fish are also high in fat content. Fresh fish, in particular, flounder, cod, halibut, perch, haddock, and sole have considerably less fat. Tuna packed in water has approximately $^1/_3$ the fat content of tuna packed in oil. Shellfish, surprisingly, although having a high cholesterol content, are low in saturated fats; however, they should be used in moderation.

POULTRY

Poultry should also be broiled or grilled, rather than fried. Discard the skin of poultry, preferably before cooking so as to avoid the saturated fats being absorbed into the carcass of the poultry. Do not use creamed sauces or gravies. Always trim off skin before eating any poultry product.

VEGETABLES

Vegetables, fortunately, are a low source of dietary fat. In many cases they can be substituted for protein because of the protein content of many vegetable products. Dried beans and peas (kidney beans, split peas, lentils and bean curd) are particularly high in fiber content and low in fat and of moderate protein value. All other vegetables and fruits are without saturated fat content and are excellent sources of carbohydrates for the body.

BAKED GOODS

Commercially prepared baked goods contain considerable saturated fat. The one exception to this is angel food cake. Sweetened fig bars, vanilla wafers and ginger-snaps have less fat than cookies and cakes made with chocolate or cream fillings. Remember to check labels for "partially hydrogenated oils." These are the so-called *trans-fats* and they can raise your blood cholesterol.

If hydrogenated or partially hydrogenated oils appear in the ingredients, you can double the amount of saturated fat listed on the label. Biscuits, muffins, croissants and butter rolls are high in fat content. English muffins, French or Italian breads are lower in fat content; however, whole-wheat, whole-grain breads are best. Bread sticks, matzos and rice cakes are low fat substitutes for most potato chips and crackers, which are high in fat content.

NOW YOU'RE COOKING WITH STEAM!

While all cooking methods decrease nutrients to some degree, the loss of vitamins, minerals, proteins, and nutritional value is considerably less with steam cooking compared to boiling. The *water-soluble vitamins* that are retained when cooking with steam are significant. Broccoli retains only 33 percent of its vitamin-C when boiled compared to 79 percent retained with steam cooking. Asparagus retains 43 percent vitamin-C compared to 78 percent when steamed; beans retain 43 percent with boiling compared to 75 percent with steam cooking. When nutrients are lost during boiling, so is the *color* and *flavor* of most foods. Steam cooking preserves the flavor whereas boiling usually disperses the flavor into the cooking water along with the nutrients.

Steam cooking is considerably *faster* than other methods of cooking and, in turn, saves considerable energy. The new type of electric steamer, which allows stacking, makes it possible to cook several different foods at one time with a considerable saving of both time and energy. The stainless steel fold-out steamer and the bamboo steamer are both inexpensive and easy to use. Fish, poultry and vegetables are excellent dishes to prepare with steam cooking. There are many excellent books and manuals on cooking with steam and they can offer you a variety of suggestions and dishes for this excellent, healthful type of food preparation.

POPCORN: THE HIGH FIBER, LOW CHOLES-TEROL, LOW CALORIE SNACK

Without the added salt, oil and butter, popcorn is probably one of the best diet snacks available. It is *low in calories and cholesterol and high in fiber.* It consequently fills you up without adding extra calories and provides the necessary fiber for the 20/20 Diet-Step® Plan. One cup of popcorn contains only 25 calories. The *electric hot-air popper* is, by far, the most efficient way to prepare popcorn. Since it uses no oil, there are no added fats and there is no cleanup necessary. These hot-air poppers can produce great quantities of popcorn in a relatively short period of time. This electric appliance is a must for your low cholesterol, high fiber walking diet. Most microwaveable popcorns contain considerable fat; however, several newer products are available in low-fat varieties. Always check the label.

There are a number of **combinations that** can be used with popcorn to add flavor and variety to this low calorie snack:

1. Popcorn can be eaten as a breakfast cereal with fruit, skim milk and a teaspoon of wheat germ.
2. Popcorn croutons: Popcorn can be used in salads and soups in place of croutons.
3. Popcorn and peanuts: Popcorn and peanuts (dry, unsalted roasted peanuts) can be an excellent evening snack with a glass of diet soda.
4. Popcorn, peanuts and raisins: Same as above.
5. Apple and popcorn: Slices of apple mixed with popcorn can be an ideal snack.
6. Cooking with popcorn: Apple popcorn crisp, chili popcorn, parmesan popcorn, garlic popcorn, peanut butter popcorn balls, raisin or cinnamon popcorn, fruit and popcorn balls are examples of serving ideas.

STAY AWAY FROM THE SCALE

Remember, no one loses weight in a straight line. When you

are on a diet, you initially lose weight, and then your weight loss levels off. This occurs even though you are eating exactly the same amount as you were when you lost the initial weight. This leveling off period or *plateau* is the single most hazardous part of any diet program. The reason is that once this plateau is reached, you begin to become discouraged and you'll say, "I'm still on the same diet but I haven't lost a pound in over a week." Discouragement leads to frustration and next you'll say, "The heck with the diet, I may as well enjoy myself and eat something I really like, since I haven't lost weight anyway." At this point 90 percent of all diets are doomed to failure since the weight loss pattern now reverses itself and becomes a *weight gain pattern.*

If you can stick out this plateau period, which incidentally is *always temporary,* you'll be surprised to see that the weight loss begins to pick up speed again. It may take a week or two at the most, but if you are patient, you will again start to lose those unwanted pounds. No one has ever satisfactorily explained this plateau period; however, physiologists believe that it is probably due to *a temporary re-adjustment of the body's metabolism* in response to the initial weight loss. No matter what the reason is, however, you will always break through the plateau period providing you don't become discouraged or frustrated. Weight loss will again resume its downward progress toward your ideal weight goal.

This plateau period is one of the main reasons that I insist that my patients do not weigh themselves daily; in fact, *weighing yourself every day is hazardous to your diet.* The reason for this is two-fold. *First,* when you weigh yourself daily and see that you are losing weight, you become happy and elated, and subconsciously you will eat to celebrate. *Secondly*, if you see that you are not losing weight as fast as you "think" you should, you become depressed and anxious, and sometime during that day you will subconsciously eat because of frustration. So, the rule of thumb is: *the more you weigh yourself the more you eat!*

Believe me, it is true. I've seen my patients go through this frustrating daily weighing process thousands of times. No one on a diet should weigh herself more than once a week, and then you will get a true measure of the effectiveness of your diet. If you must weigh yourself, then Wednesday is the best day to weigh yourself each week. Monday and Friday are the worst days for weighing in, since they follow and precede the weekend and lead to frustrating eating binges. It took a long time to gain all that weight; you can't take it off overnight. Be patient!

DIET TIPS FOR SLIM HIPS

1. Don't skip meals

Skipping meals lowers your blood sugar, which brings on cravings for high-carbohydrate, high-calorie foods. In many people, going hungry can bring on "hunger headaches" similar to migraine-type headaches. Eating 3-4 even 5 small meals per day is far superior to eating one or two large meals. If your blood sugar remains constant, then you're less likely to overeat and gain weight.

Have you ever noticed thin wiry women who seem to be eating all the time but never get fat? That's because they eat small, frequent meals which are lower in calories, and their metabolism seems to burn them up at a faster rate, rather than having to deal with a large number of calories all at once. And besides, small, frequent meals are usually consumed by active rather than sedentary people. The high-calorie, large-meal eater usually eats and sits and sits and eats. And when she is finished eating, she sits some more, because she's too bloated to get up and move around. The small meal eater is up and about before you know it.

2. Eliminate the fat in your diet

Most people do not realize the amount of fat calories that they consume each day. The first order of business is to find the fat in your diet and eliminate it. Everyone knows that there's fat in bacon, lunchmeats, eggs, butter, ice cream, milk and cheese. But not everyone realizes that there's considerable fat in donuts, cakes, pies, muffins, margarine, mayonnaise, chicken and tuna salad, coffee creamers, yogurt, cream cheese and cottage cheese -- (even the ones marked low-fat).

Your body metabolizes fats and carbohydrates together in a set ratio governed genetically by your individual body's metabolism. When you restrict the number of fat calories that you consume, then your body's metabolism automatically controls the amount of refined carbohydrate calories that you actually eat. By restricting the fat calories eaten you crave less refined carbohydrates in your diet. The combination of less fat eaten combined with less refined carbohydrates craved, makes it next to impossible for you to put on excess weight. So when you *eat less fat you're less likely to get fat.* Sounds simple? It is! That's one of the ways that the Diet-Step®: 20 Grams Fat/20 Grams Fiber works.

3. Avoid eating fast and fast-food eating

If you're a fast eater or a fast-food eater -- watch out! When you consume food at a rapid pace, you have a greater tendency to consume excess calories by overeating. The reason for this is that it takes 15-20 minutes for the brain's appetite regulator (the appestat) to receive the signals that your body's stomach is full. If you eat your meal rapidly in 5 or 10 minutes as you often do in fast-food restaurants, then your appestat will never know that you've eaten. Subsequently, you'll still be as hungry as you were before you wolfed down that bacon double-cheese burger. And you'll probably order a milk-shake and a large order of french fries. By the time you get those down the hatch your brain will just be receiving the first signals that you're full from the original double bacon-cheese burger that you ate in the first 5 minutes. Well, it's too late by then. The appestat will never know that you've eaten 620 calories and 38 grams of fat (bacon double cheeseburger), and 590 calories and 30 grams of fat (large french fries), and 400 calories and 9 grams of fat (milk-shake). Only your waistline, hips and thighs will be the wiser.

4. Chew food thoroughly and eat foods that need chewing

Foods that require a good bit of chewing like apples, corn, celery, carrots, salads, cucumber, raw vegetables (cauliflower, broccoli, string beans, radishes, etc) are excellent diet foods since they take time to chew and consequently, the brain's appetite regulating mechanism (appestat) is satisfied long before you've had a chance to consume too many calories.

An apple a day not only keeps the doctor away, but it also keeps the fat away from your body. Apples are high-fiber foods which not only take longer to eat than most other comparably sized-foods, but have many nutritional advantages over low-fiber foods. One reason the appestat is appeased early is the time that it takes you to eat an apple. The other reason is that the high-fiber content of apples and similar high-fiber foods produces more bulk in the stomach, making you feel full faster.

5. Don't skip breakfast

People who never eat breakfast usually make up for it sometime during the day and then some. By the time lunch comes your low blood sugar gives you a ravenous appetite and you're sure to overeat. Or you may get hungry long before lunch time arrives and you'll end up stuffing donuts and coffee into your face. Remember, too, that caffeine is an appetite stimulant, and you should be careful not to drink too much coffee or tea. People who skip breakfast seem to make up for it three-fold by snacking mid-morning, mid-afternoon and late evening. This appears to be due to the fact that the metabolism seems to slow down later in the day in non-breakfast eaters. The body reacts to a lack of breakfast as if it is trying to starve itself, and so it slows down your metabolism to keep you from starving to death. This results in sluggishness and fatigue which in turn causes you to "just eat something" in order to feel better. Eating speeds up the metabolism, and elevates the blood sugar, and lo-and-behold, you feel better. Then the blood sugar rapidly drops again and you feel fatigued again and so you eat again. This is called *functional hypoglycemia* or low blood sugar, which results from just skipping meals. Other causes of hypoglycemia are the result of excess alcohol, caffeine, nicotine, sugar and stress.

6. Dieting can be fun!

The most important part of any successful diet is starting it. Once you've made up your mind to begin your diet you're half way there. You must also be able to have fun with your diet. The Diet-Step®: 20 Grams Fat/20 Grams Fiber Diet does not require much discipline, since it's easy to follow and you see results quickly. In fact, the diet is fun to follow, since you know you are losing weight, by eating healthful, colorful, exciting, good-tasting foods. Try some, it's fun!

7. Healthy foods like you!

Foods that are good for you are also good for your figure. Most of the foods that promote good health are also foods that help you stay slim and trim.

Fruits - are high in fiber and low in calories. They fill you up without filling you out. Fruits satisfy the appestat by taking longer to consume and they promote good bowel health by providing adequate fiber, which in turn also reduces your appetite. Fruits are not only low-fat, low-calorie foods, but they are especially rich in *potassium*. Potassium is an essential element, which appears to have blood pressure lowering properties. In a recent medical study, potassium-rich foods reduced the risk of strokes by more than 30% in individuals who had known hypertension.

Fruits are also good sources of pectin, a fiber found in many fruits and vegetables. This particular type of fiber helps to lower blood cholesterol. Many of these fruits, which are high in pectin, also contain vitamin C, which helps the pectin lower cholesterol even more than pectin alone. Vitamin C also is important in boosting our immune system and also has cancer-inhibiting factors built into its structure. Some of the fruits that are rich in both pectin and vitamin C are oranges, pears, grapefruit, bananas, berries, apples and tangerines. Fruits are also high in phyto-nutrients, which can help to prevent many types of cancers and heart disease.

Fish - Studies show that diets rich in fish lower blood pressure 15-20% in hypertensive men. A study conducted at the Cardiovascular Research Institute in West Germany showed that men with mild hypertension who ate 3 cans of mackerel per week had a significant reduction in their blood pressures. Other studies in the United States have confirmed these findings.

Fish oil has been shown to reduce blood fats, and consequently, slow the formation of deposits of cholesterol in the arteries. In a study at the University of Chicago, monkeys on a diet high in fish oil developed less cholesterol deposits in their arteries than monkeys fed a diet high in saturated fat and coconut oil. The monkeys fed fish oil also had lower total cholesterol and LDL cholesterol levels than the monkeys fed the high saturated fat diet. Another study conducted at Harvard Medical School appears to indicate that fish-oils also have a cancer-inhibiting factor. In a study of rats with breast cancer, fish-oils seem to slow the spread of the disease significantly more than diets high in saturated fat or poly-unsaturated fats and even more than just a low-fat diet.

It appears that the omega-3 fatty acids present in fish oils is the ingredient responsible for the cholesterol-lowering and cancer-inhibiting effects. Fish is not only low in saturated fat and calories but it's high in omega-3 fatty acids that help to lower both your cholesterol and triglyceride levels. Eat fish 2-3 times per week for a healthy heart and a slim body. Many recent studies at major universities have also found that the omega-3 oils help to prevent platelet cells in the blood from getting sticky, decreasing the tendency for blood clots to form. Eskimos and the Japanese who consume lots of fish don't typically have heart attacks from fat-clogged arteries.

Omega-3 fatty acids found in fish oil also have been found to be essential for brain function. Recent studies have found that a lack of omega-3 fatty acids may be responsible for learning disabilities, memory loss, difficulty concentrating and certain degenerative diseases, including Alzheimer's disease. In a recent study, age-related memory decline was halted or slowed down considerably in women who ate ¾ oz. of fish every other day. New evidence has also shown that fish oils may even help in the treatment of major depression and other neurologic and psychiatric disorders.

Cereal grains, especially, oats and bran: Provide water-soluble fiber that helps to lower both cholesterol and triglyceride levels. These high fiber cereals also promote good bowel health by reducing constipation and preventing hemorrhoids, diverticulitis, appendicitis, varicose veins and reducing the incidence of colon cancer.

Fowl: Lean white meat of turkey and chicken is low in calories and fat, promoting good health and a slim figure. Make sure you remove the skin, which contains high amounts of saturated fat, before eating fowl.

Onion, garlic and peppers: Help to lower levels of blood fats, lower blood pressure and help to make the blood less likely to clot. These foods contain certain natural chemical substances that actually thin your blood.

Vegetables: It's important to eat more vegetables of the cabbage-family, particularly broccoli, cauliflower, spinach, brussels sprouts, and squash. These foods are not only high in fiber but they are also high in both vitamins A and C, and are rich in phyto-nutrients, which are cancer-fighting agents.

Many vegetables also rich in potassium are sweet potatoes, potatoes, squash, spinach, beets, tomatoes and green peppers. Boiling destroys more than 35-40% of the potassium in vegetables, so remember to eat more raw vegetables and steam or microwave vegetables rather than boil them, in order to reduce potassium loss.

Carrots and leafy green vegetables contain beta-carotene and other carotenes, which are chemical pre-cursors to vitamin A. Beta-carotene is converted to vitamin A in the body. Vitamin A inhibits compounds called free-radicals in the body, which may cause normal cells to turn cancerous. Vitamin A also maintains the integrity of the lining of the lungs and the intestinal tract. Beta-carotene appears to have a protective effect against both lung and colon cancer. A recent study conducted at the New York State University in Buffalo found that people with lung cancer had significantly lower blood levels of beta-carotene than a similar number of people who were free of the disease. Similar studies have shown that patients with colon cancer also have lower levels of beta-carotene than a comparable number of healthy individuals.

DIETS JUST DON'T WORK!

Consumer Reports polled 95,000 subscribers who tried to lose weight over the last 3-5 years. Over 19,000 subscribers used commercially supervised diet programs and the rest tried to lose weight on their own. The results of both groups were similar in that dieters lost an average of 10 - 12 pounds while on their respective diets. The discouraging news, however, is that most of the respondents to this survey regained almost half of their weight loss in the first 3 - 6 months after ending the diet program and 2/3 of the weight was regained in 2 years. Only 20% of these dieters were able to keep off 2/3 of the weight they had lost for more than a 2-year period.

Many of these commercial diet programs cost an average of $65 - 70 per week - a pretty hefty price to pay for a temporary weight loss plan.

The diet business, ranging from diet centers, spas, health clubs and diet foods, generated more than 35 billion dollars in revenues in 1999. That figure is comparable to the casino industry, both of which are just different forms of gambling. It's time that women take control of their diet programs as well as control over their wallets. There is no need to spend hard-earned money on inefficient diet plans when there's a free, easy, effective plan that you can follow for the rest of your life. And best of all, it works. There's no rebound weight gain, and you're not locked into buying specially prepared foods (dehydrated or otherwise) or attending pep--rally meetings every week. The schedule you follow is your own life's schedule, which, as you know, is difficult enough for you to juggle without any complicated diet program.

Yes, we're talking about <u>Diet-Step®: 20 Grams/20 Minutes: For Women Only!</u> As you've seen in Chapter 2 (<u>Diet-Step®: 20 Grams Fat/20 Grams Fiber)</u>, you can lose weight easily and quickly with a minimum of effort on your part. What's more, the weight stays off permanently. As you'll see in the next section on the <u>Fit-Step® plan,</u> you'll be able to: 1. Achieve and maintain cardiovascular fitness; 2. Build a fitter, trimmer you; 3. Sculpt and mold your body beautifully; 4. Look younger and live longer; 5. And have fun to boot -- <u>all in just 20 minutes a day.</u> Sound easy? It is!

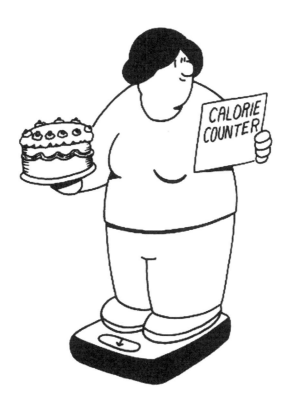

**"I HAVE A WEIGHT PROBLEM--I CAN'T WAIT
FOR DESSERT!"**

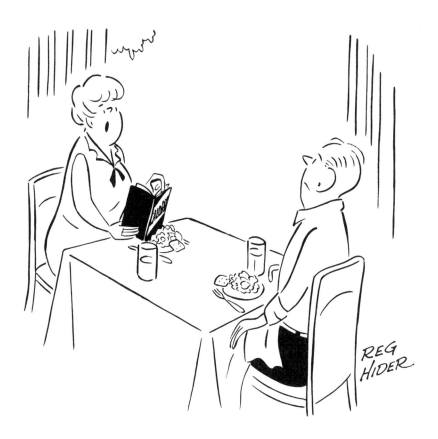

"COUNTING CALORIES MAKES ME HUNGRY."

CHAPTER 6

FAT & FIBER COUNTER
****
Sources of Information

- United States Department of Agriculture
- Center for Science and Public Interest
- Food Manufacturers, Processors and Distributors
- Bowes and Church's Food Values of Portions Commonly Used (Pennington and Church, 17th Ed.)
- Scientific Journals and Publications
- Author Extrapolations

Interpreting Food Labels

- Sugar Free: Less than $1/2$ gram sugar per serving
- Calorie Free: No more than 5 calories per serving
- Salt Free: Less than 5 milligrams of sodium per serving
- Low Sodium: No more than 140 milligrams of sodium per serving
- Fat Free: Less than $1/2$ gram fat per serving
- Low Fat: No more than 3 grams fat per serving
- Reduced Fat: At least 25% less fat than comparison food
- Low Saturated Fat: No more than 1 gram saturated fat per serving
- Reduced Saturated Fat: No more than 50% saturated fat of comparison food
- Light: 1/2 the fat in or 1/3 fewer calories than the regular version of a similar food

Fat and Fiber Chart

	Serving	Tot. Fat (g)	Sat. Fat (g)	Chol. (mg)	Fiber (g)
BREADS AND FLOUR					
bagel, plain	1 medium	1.1	0.2	0	2
bagel, cinnamon raisin	1 medium	1.2	0.2	0	2
barley flour	1 cup	0.5	1.3	0	3
biscuit					
plain	1 medium	6.6	1.9	3	1
buttermilk	1 medium	5.8	0.9	2	1
from mix	1 medium	4.3	1.2	3	1
bread					
cracked wheat	1 slice	1.0	0.2	0	1
French/Vienna	1 slice	1.0	0.2	0	1
Italian	1 slice	0.5	0.1	0	1
matzoh	1 piece	0.5	0.1	0	0
mixed grain	1 slice	0.9	0.2	0	2
multigrain, "lite"	1 slice	0.5	0.0	2	3
pita, plain	1 large	0.7	0.1	0	2
pita, whole wheat	1 large	1.2	0.3	0	4
pumpernickel	1 slice	0.8	0.0	0	2
raisin	1 slice	1.1	0.3	0	1
rye	1 slice	0.9	0.2	0	2
sourdough	1 slice	0.8	0.2	0	1
wheat, commercial	1 slice	1.1	0.3	0	2
wheat, "lite"	1 slice	0.5	0.1	0	3
white, commercial	1 slice	1.0	0.2	0	0
white, "lite"	1 slice	0.5	0.1	0	1
whole wheat, commercial	1 slice	1.2	0.3	0	3
breadcrumbs	1 cup	1.5	1.3	0	2
breadsticks	2 small	0.5	0.2	0	0
bulgar	1/2 cup	2.0	0.3	0	5.2
cornbread	1 piece	5.5	2.0	12	1.5
cornflake crumbs	1 oz.	0.0	0.0	0	1
cornmeal, dry	1/2 cup	2.3	0.3	0	6
cornstarch	1 T	0.0	0.0	0	0
crackers					
cheese	5 pieces	4.9	1.6	4	0
Cheese Nips	13 crackers	3.2	1.2	3	0
cheese w/peanut butter	2 oz. Pkg.	13.5	2.9	7	1
Goldfish, any flavor	12 crackers	2.0	0.7	1	0
graham	2 squares	1.3	0.4	0	0
Harvest Wheats	4 crackers	3.6	1.1	0	1
melba toast	1 piece	0.2	0.0	0	0
oyster	15 crackers	2.1	0.3	0	0

	Serving	Tot. Fat (g)	Sat. Fat (g)	Chol. (mg)	Fiber (g)
rice cakes	1 piece	0.2	0.0	0	0
Ritz	3 crackers	3.0	1.1	1	0
Ritz cheese	3 crackers	3.9	1.4	2	0
Ryekrisp, plain	2 crackers	0.2	0.0	0	2
Ryekrisp, sesame	2 crackers	1.4	0.4	0	3
saltines	2 crackers	0.7	0.1	0	0
sesame wafers	3 crackers	3.0	0.8	0	0
Snackwell's wheat	5 crackers	0.0	0.0	0	1
Sociables	6 crackers	3.0	1.1	0	0
soda	5 crackers	1.9	0.3	0	0
toasted w/peanut butter	1.5 oz. Pkg.	10.5	2.9	2	0
Triscuit	2 crackers	1.6	0.3	0	1
Vegetable Thins	7 crackers	4.0	1.0	0	0
Wheat Thins	4 crackers	1.5	0.6	0	0
wheat w/cheese	1.5 oz. Pkg.	10.9	2.8	1	0
crepe	1 medium	12.5	4.1	37	0
croissant	1 medium	11.5	6.9	30	1
croutons, commercial	1/4 cup	1.8	0.5	0	1
Danish pastry	1 medium	19.3	6.8	30	1
doughnut					
cake	(1) 2 oz.	16.2	4.1	24	1
yeast	(1) 2 oz.	13.3	5.2	21	1
English muffin					
plain	1	1.1	0.2	0	1
w/raisins	1	1.2	0.2	0	1
whole wheat	1	2.0	0.5	0	2
flour					
buckwheat	1 cup	3.0	0.7	0	8
rice	1 cup	1.3	0.5	0	3
rye	1 cup	2.2	0.2	0	11
soy	1 cup	16.0	2.5	0	4
white, all purpose	1 cup	1.2	0.2	0	4
whole wheat	1 cup	2.3	0.4	0	12
French toast					
frzn variety	1 slice	6.0	1.0	54	0
hmde	1 slice	10.7	2.6	75	1
funnel cake	4 in. diam.	12.8	2.5	48	1
muffins					
banana nut	1 medium	5.0	2.2	20	2
blueberry, from mix	1 medium	5.1	1.1	9	1
bran, hmde	1 medium	5.8	1.2	16	3
corn	1 medium	4.8	0.9	18	2

	Serving	Tot. Fat (g)	Sat. Fat (g)	Chol. (mg)	Fiber (g)
white, plain	1 medium	5.4	1.1	12	1
pancakes					
blueberry, from mix	3 medium	15.0	4.3	80	4
buckwheat, from mix	3 medium	12.3	3.9	75	3
buttermilk, from mix	3 medium	10.0	3.2	80	2
"lite," from mix	3 medium	2.0	0.6	20	5
whole wheat, from mix	3 medium	3.0	1.0	30	6
phyllo dough	2 oz.	6.4	0.5	0	1
pie crust, plain	1/8 pie	8.0	1.9	0	0
popover	1	5.0	2.6	51	0
rice bran	1 oz.	0.4	0.1	0	2
rolls					
crescent	1	5.6	2.8	6	1
croissant	1 small	6.0	3.5	21	0
French	1	0.4	0.1	0	1
hamburger	1	3.0	0.8	1	1
hard	1	1.2	0.3	1	1
hot dog	1	2.1	0.5	1	1
kaiser	1 medium	2.0	0.5	0	0
raisin	1 large	1.9	0.5	0	1
rye, dark	1	1.6	0.1	0	2
rye, light, hard	1	1.0	0.1	0	2
sandwich	1	3.1	0.4	2	1
sesame seed	1	2.1	0.6	1	1
sourdough	1	1.0	0.0	0	1
submarine/hoagie	1 medium	3.0	0.8	3	2
wheat	1	1.7	0.4	0	1
white, commercial	1	2.2	1.0	1	0
whole wheat	1	1.1	0.2	1	3
scone	1	5.5	1.5	28	1
soft pretzel	1 medium	1.5	0.7	2	1.5
stuffing					
bread, from mix	1/2 cup	12.2	6.0	0	0
cornbread, from mix	1/2 cup	4.8	2.5	43	0
Stove Top	1/2 cup	9.0	5.0	21	0
sweet roll, iced	1 medium	7.9	2.1	20	1
toaster pastry	1	5.0	0.8	0	0
tortilla					
corn (unfried)	1 medium	1.1	0.2	0	1
flour	1 medium	2.5	1.1	0	1
turnover, fruit filled	1	15.0	3.7	0	1
waffle					

	Serving	Total Fat (g)	Sat. Fat (g)	Chol. (mg)	Fiber (g)
frozen	1 medium	3.2	0.8	11	1
hmde	1 medium	9.5	4.1	50	1
from mix	1 medium	8.5	3.0	48	1
CEREALS					
All Bran	1/3 cup	0.5	0.1	0	10
Apple Jacks	1 cup	0.1	0.0	0	1
Bran, 100%	1/2 cup	1.9	0.3	0	9
Bran Chex	1 cup	1.2	0.2	0	9
Bran Flakes, 40%	1 cup	0.7	0.1	0	6
Cheerios	1 cup	1.6	0.3	0	2
Cocoa Krispies	1 cup	0.5	0.2	0	0
Corn Chex	1 cup	0.1	0.0	0	1
cornflakes	1 cup	0.1	0.0	0	1
Cracklin' Oat Bran	1/3 cup	2.7	1.3	0	3
Cream of Wheat w/o added fat	1/2 cup	0.3	0.0	0	0
Crispix	1 cup	0.0	0.0	0	1
Fiber One	1 cup	2.2	0.4	0	13
Frosted Bran, Kellogg's	3/4 cup	0.0	0.0	0	3
Frosted Mini-Wheats	4 biscuits	0.3	0.0	0	1
Fruit & Fibre w/dates, raisins,					
walnuts	2/3 cup	2.0	0.3	0	5
w/peaches, almonds	2/3 cup	2.0	0.3	0	5
Fruitful Bran	2/3 cup	0.0	0.0	0	5
Fruit Loops	1 cup	0.5	0.0	0	1
Golden Grahams	3/4 cup	1.1	0.1	0	1
granola					
commercial brands	1/3 cup	4.9	1.8	0	3
low-fat, Kellogg's	1/3 cup	2.0	0.0	0	2
Grapenut Flakes	1 cup	0.4	0.2	0	2
Grapenuts	1/4 cup	0.1	0.0	0	2
Life, plain or cinn.	1 cup	2.5	0.5	0	4
Mueslix, Kellogg's	1/2 cup	1.0	0.8	0	5
Nutri-Grain, Kellogg's					
almond raisin	2/3 cup	2.0	0.4	0	3
raisin bran	1 cup	1.0	0.1	0	5
wheat	2/3 cup	0.3	0.0	0	3
oat bran, cooked cereal					
w/o added fat	1/2 cup	0.5	0.1	0	2
oats					
instant	1 packet	1.7	0.2	0	1
w/o added fat	1/2 cup	1.2	0.2	0	1
Product 19	1 cup	0.2	0.0	0	1

	Serving	Total Fat (g)	Sat. Fat (g)	Chol. (mg)	Fiber (g)
puffed rice	1 cup	0.2	0.0	0	1
puffed wheat	1 cup	0.1	0.0	0	1
Raisin Bran	1 cup	0.8	0.1	0	5
Rice Chex	1 cup	0.1	0.0	0	1
Rice Krispies	1 cup	0.2	0.0	0	0
shredded wheat	1 cup	0.3	0.0	0	2
Special K	1 cup	0.1	0.0	0	0
Sugar Frosted Flakes	1 cup	0.5	0.1	0	1
Total	1 cup	0.7	0.1	0	2
Total raisin bran	1 cup	1.0	0.1	0	5
Wheat Chex	1 cup	1.2	0.2	0	6
Wheaties	1 cup	0.5	0.1	0	2
DAIRY PRODUCTS					
cheeses					
American					
processed	1 oz.	8.9	5.6	27	0
reduced calorie	1 oz.	2.0	1.0	12	0
blue	1 oz.	8.2	5.3	21	0
Borden's Fat Free	1 oz.	<0.5	<0.3	<5	0
Borden's Lite Line	1 oz.	2.0	<1.0	NA	0
caraway	1 oz.	8.3	5.4	30	0
cheddar	1 oz.	9.2	5.0	26	0
cheese sauce	1/4 cup	9.8	4.3	20	0
cheese spread, Kraft	1 oz.	6.0	3.8	16	0
Cheez Whiz	1 oz.	6.0	3.1	16	0
cottage cheese					
1% fat	1/2 cup	1.2	0.8	5	0
2% fat	1/2 cup	2.2	1.4	10	0
creamed	1/2 cup	5.1	3.2	17	0
cream cheese					
Kraft Free	1 oz. (2T)	0.0	0.0	5	0
lite	1 oz. (2T)	6.6	4.2	20	0
regular	1 oz. (2T)	9.9	6.2	31	0
Edam	1 oz.	7.9	5.0	25	0
feta	1 oz.	6.0	4.2	25	0
Gouda	1 oz.	7.8	5.0	32	0
Jarlsberg	1 oz.	6.9	4.2	16	0
Kraft American Singles	1 oz.	7.5	4.3	25	0
Kraft Free Singles	1 oz.	0.0	0.0	5	0
Kraft Light Singles	1 oz.	4.0	2.0	15	0
Light n' Lively singles	1 oz.	4.0	2.0	15	0
Monterey Jack	1 oz.	8.6	5.0	30	0

	Serving	Total Fat (g)	Sat. Fat (g)	Chol. (mg)	Fiber (g)
mozzarella					
part skim	1 oz.	4.5	2.4	16	0
whole milk	1 oz.	6.1	3.7	22	0
Muenster	1 oz.	8.5	5.4	27	0
Parmesan					
grated	1 T	1.5	1.0	4	0
hard	1 oz.	7.3	4.7	19	0
pimento cheese spread	1 oz.	8.9	5.6	27	0
provolone	1 oz.	7.6	4.8	20	0
ricotta					
"lite" reduced fat	1/2 cup	4.0	2.4	15	0
part skim	1/2 cup	9.8	6.1	38	0
whole milk	1/2 cup	16.1	10.3	63	0
Romano	1 oz.	7.6	4.9	29	0
Roquefort	1 oz.	7.8	5.0	24	0
Swiss					
Alpine Lace	1 oz.	1.5	0.5	5	0
sliced	1oz.	7.8	5.0	26	0
Velveeta	1 oz.	7.0	4.0	20	0
Velveeta Light	1 oz.	4.0	2.0	15	0
Eggs					
boiled-poached	1	5.6	1.6	213	0
fried w/ 1/2 t margarine	1 large	7.6	2.7	240	0
omelet					
2 oz. cheese, 3 egg	1	37.0	12.3	480	0
plain, 3 egg	1	21.3	5.2	430	0
Spanish, 2 egg	1	18.0	5.9	375	1
scrambled w/milk	1 large	8.0	2.8	214	0
substitute, frzn	1/4 cup	0.0	0.0	0	0
white	1 large	0.0	0.0	0	0
yolk	1 large	5.6	1.6	213	0
Milk and Yogurt					
buttermilk					
1% fat	1 cup	2.2	1.3	9	0
dry	1 T	0.4	0.2	5	0
choc. milk					
2% fat	1 cup	5.0	3.1	17	0
whole	1 cup	8.5	5.3	30	0
evaporated milk					
skim	1/2 cup	0.4	0.0	0	0
whole	1/2 cup	9.5	5.8	37	0
hot cocoa					

	Serving	Total Fat (g)	Sat. Fat (g)	Chol. (mg)	Fiber (g)
mix w/water	1 cup	3.0	0.7	5	0
w/skim milk	1 cup	2.0	0.9	12	0
w/whole milk	1 cup	9.1	5.6	33	0
low fat milk					
1/2% fat	1 cup	1.0	4.0	10	0
1% fat	1 cup	2.6	1.6	10	0
2% fat	1 cup	4.7	2.9	18	0
milkshake					
choc. thick	1 cup	6.1	3.8	24	1
vanilla, thick	1 cup	6.9	4.3	27	0
skim milk					
liquid	1 cup	0.4	0.3	4	0
nonfat dry powder	1/4 cup	0.2	0.2	6	0
whole milk					
3.5% fat	1 cup	8.2	5.0	34	0
dry powder	1/4 cup	8.6	5.4	31	0
yogurt					
frzn, low fat	1/2 cup	3.0	2.0	10	0
frzn, nonfat	1/2 cup	0.2	0.0	0	0
fruit flavored, low fat	1 cup	2.6	0.1	10	0
plain					
low fat	1 cup	3.5	2.3	14	0
skim (nonfat)	1 cup	0.4	0.3	4	0
whole milk	1 cup	7.4	4.8	29	0
DESSERTS					
apple betty	1/2 cup	13.3	2.7	0	3
baklava	1 piece	29.2	7.2	7	2
brownie					
choc., plain	1	5.0	1.5	14	0
choc. w/frosting	1	9.0	1.5	20	1
choc. w/nuts	1	7.3	1.8	10	1
cake					
angel food	1/8 cake	0.1	0.0	0	0
banana	1/8 cake	14.5	2.5	50	1
black forest	1/8 cake	15.0	2.0	50	1
carrot w/frosting	1/8 cake	18.0	3.6	53	3
choc. w/frosting	1/8 cake	16.0	4.0	77	2
coconut w/frosting	1/8 cake	17.0	5.4	51	2
coffee cake	1/8 cake	6.1	1.0	42	1
devil's food, "light," from mix	1/8 cake	2.8	1.1	42	0
German choc. w/frosting	1/8 cake	17.0	4.1	72	2
gingerbread	1/8 cake	2.6	0.9	1.3	0

	Serving	Total Fat (g)	Sat. Fat (g)	Chol. (mg)	Fiber (g)
lemon chiffon	1/8 cake	3.0	0.7	3	0
marble w/frosting	1/8 cake	15.0	2.5	62	1
pound	1/8 cake	8.2	4.0	50	1
spice w/frosting	1/8 cake	10.2	2.8	48	1
sponge	1/8 cake	2.0	0.5	50	0
white w/frosting	1/8 cake	13.1	3.0	30	1
white, "light," from mix	1/8 cake	2.6	0.5	15	0
yellow, "light," from mix	1/8 cake	3.0	1.2	35	0
yellow w/frosting	1/8 cake	14.0	4.0	50	1
cheesecake, traditional	1/8 pie	22.0	10.4	36	0
cobbler					
w/biscuit topping	1/2 cup	6.0	1.7	2	3
w/pie-crust topping	1/2 cup	9.3	3.6	5	3
cookie					
animal	15 cookies	4.7	1.2	0	0
Chantilly, Pepperidge Farm	1	2.0	1.0	<5	0
choc.	1	3.3	1.0	6	0
choc. chip hmde	1	3.7	2.0	8	0
choc. chip, Pepperidge Farm	1	2.5	1.4	<5	0
choc. sandwich (Oreo type)	1	2.1	0.4	0	0
Entenmann's fat-free	2	0.0	0.0	0	0
fat-free Newtons	1	0.0	0.0	0	0
fig bar	1	1.0	0.2	0	1
Fig Newtons	1	1.0	0.3	0	0
gingersnap	1	1.6	0.3	0	0
graham cracker, choc. covered	1	3.1	0.9	0	0
macaroon, coconut	1	3.4	1.3	0	0
oatmeal	1	3.2	0.6	0	0
oatmeal raisin	1	3.0	0.8	0	0
peanut butter	1	3.2	1.0	6	1
Rice Krispie Bar	1	0.9	0.3	0	0
shortbread	1	2.3	0.4	2	0
cupcake					
choc. w/icing	1	5.5	2.1	22	1
yellow w/icing	1	6.0	2.3	23	1
custard, baked	1/2 cup	6.9	3.4	123	0
date bar	1 bar	2.0	0.7	2	1
dumpling, fruit	1 piece	15.1	5.5	8	2
éclair (with choc. icing & custard	1 small	15.4	5.7	115	0
fruitcake	1 piece	6.2	1.4	11	1
fruit ice, Italian	1/2 cup	0.0	0.0	0	0
Fudgesicle	1 bar	0.4	0.2	3	1

	Serving	Total Fat (g)	Sat. Fat (g)	Chol. (mg)	Fiber (g)
granola bar	1 bar	6.8	1.5	0	1
ice cream					
choc. (10% fat)	1/2 cup	7.3	4.5	23	1
choc. (16% fat)	1/2 cup	17.0	8.9	44	0
dietetic, sugar-free	1/2 cup	3.5	1.3	27	0
vanilla soft serve	1/2 cup	11.3	6.4	76	0
strawberry (10% fat)	1/2 cup	6.0	4.0	28	0
vanilla (10% fat)	1/2 cup	7.0	5.4	28	0
vanilla (16% fat)	1/2 cup	11.9	7.4	44	0
ice cream bar					
choc. coated	1 bar	11.5	10.0	23	0
toffee crunch	1 bar	10.2	7.0	9	1
ice cream cake roll	1 slice	6.9	4.0	52	0
ice cream cone (cone only)	1 medium	0.3	0.1	0	0
ice cream drumstick	1	10.0	4.1	14	1
ice cream sandwich	1	8.3	4.4	12	0
ice milk					
choc.	1/2 cup	2.0	1.3	9	0
soft serve, all flavors	1/2 cup	2.3	1.4	7	0
strawberry	1/2 cup	2.5	1.2	7	0
vanilla	1/2 cup	2.8	1.5	8	0
jello	1/2 cup	0.0	0.0	0	0
ladyfinger	1	2.0	0.5	80	0
lemon bars	1 bar	3.2	7.0	13	0
mousse, choc.	1/2 cup	15.5	8.7	124	1
napolean	1 piece	5.3	2.6	10	0
pie					
apple	1/8 pie	16.9	2.3	3	3
banana cream or custard	1/8 pie	14.0	10.0	35	1
blueberry	1/8 pie	17.3	4.0	0	3
Boston cream pie	1/8 pie	10.0	3.1	20	1
cherry	1/8 pie	18.1	5.0	0	2
choc. cream	1/8 pie	13.0	4.5	15	3
coconut cream or custard	1/8 pie	19.0	7.0	80	1
key lime	1/8 pie	19.0	6.8	10	1
lemon chiffon	1/8 pie	13.5	3.7	15	1
lemon meringue, traditional	1/8 pie	13.1	5.1	50	1
peach	1/8 pie	17.7	4.6	3	3
pecan	1/8 pie	23.0	3.5	100	2
pumpkin	1/8 pie	16.8	5.7	109	
raisin	1/8 pie	12.9	3.1	0	1
rhubarb	1/8 pie	17.1	4.5	2	3

	Serving	Total Fat (g)	Sat. Fat (g)	Chol. (mg)	Fiber (g)
strawberry	1/8 pie	9.1	4.5	2	1
sweet potato	1/8 pie	18.2	6.0	70	2
pie tart, fruit filled	1	18.7	6.2	23	2
Popsicle	1 bar	0.0	0.0	0	0
pudding					
any flavor except choc.	1/2 cup	4.3	2.5	70	0
bread w/raisins	1/2 cup	7.4	2.9	78	1
choc. w/whole milk	1/2 cup	5.7	3.1	17	1
from mix w/skim milk	1/2 cup	0.0	0.0	0	0
rice w/whole milk	1/2 cup	4.4	2.5	16	1
sugar free varieties	1/2 cup	2.2	1.4	10	0
tapioca, w/2% milk	1/2 cup	2.4	1.5	8	0
pudding pop, frzn	1 bar	2.0	1.0	2	0
sherbert	1/2 cup	1.0	0.5	7	0
souffle, choc	1/2 cup	3.9	1.4	42	0
strudel, fruit	1/2 cup	1.2	0.1	2	1
toppings					
butterscotch/caramel	3 T	0.1	0.0	0	0
cherry	3 T	0.1	0.0	0	0
choc. fudge	2 T	4.0	2.0	0	0
choc. syrup, Hershey	2 T	0.4	0.2	0	0
marshmallow	3 T	0.0	0.0	0	0
milk choc. fudge	2 T	5.0	2.9	5	0
pecans in syrup	3 T	2.8	1.1	0	2
pineapple	3 T	0.2	0.0	0	0
strawberry	3 T	0.1	0.0	0	0
whipped topping					
aerosol	1/4 cup	3.6	1.4	0	0
from mix	1/4 cup	2.0	1.2	4	0
frzn, tub	1/4 cup	4.8	3.6	0	0
non-fat	1 T	0.0	0.0	0	0
whipping cream					
heavy, fluid	1 T	5.6	3.5	21	0
light, fluid	1 T	4.6	2.9	17	0
turnover, fruit filled	1	19.3	5.4	2	1
yogurt, frozen					
low fat	1/2 cup	1.9	1.2	10	0
nonfat	1/2 cup	0.0	0.0	0	0
CANDY					
butterscotch					
candy	6 pieces	1.3	0.4	0	0
chips	1 oz.	8.3	6.8	0	0

	Serving	Total Fat (g)	Sat. Fat (g)	Chol. (mg)	Fiber (g)
candied fruit					
apricot	1 oz.	0.1	0.0	0	1
cherry	1 oz.	0.1	0.0	0	1
citrus peel	1 oz.	0.1	0.0	0	1
figs	1 oz.	0.1	0.0	0	2
candy bar (average)	1 oz.	8.5	4.5	5	1
caramels					
plain or choc. w/nuts	1 oz.	4.6	2.2	10	0
plain or choc. w/o nuts	1 oz.	3.0	1.3	9	0
choc.-covered cherries	1 oz.	4.9	2.9	1	1
choc.-covered cream center	1 oz.	4.9	2.6	1	1
choc.-covered mint patty	1 small	1.5	0.8	0	0
choc.-covered peanuts	1 oz.	11.7	4.6	0	2
choc.-covered raisins	1 oz.	4.9	2.9	3	1
choc. kisses	6 pieces	9.0	5.0	6	1
choc. stars	6 pieces	8.1	4.7	5	1
Cracker Jack	1 cup	3.3	0.4	0	2
English toffee	1 oz.	2.8	1.7	5	0
fudge					
choc.	1 oz.	3.4	1.5	1	0
choc. w/nuts	1 oz.	4.9	1.2	1	0
gumdrops	28 pieces	0.2	0.0	0	0
Gummy Bears	1 oz.	0.1	0.0	0	0
hard candy	6 pieces	0.3	0.0	0	0
jelly beans	1 oz.	0.0	0.0	0	0
licorice	1 oz.	0.1	0.0	0	0
Life Savers	5 pieces	0.1	0.0	0	0
M&M's					
choc. only	1 oz.	5.6	2.4	3	1
peanut	1 oz.	7.8	2.4	4	1
malted-milk balls	1 oz.	7.1	4.2	3	1
marshmallow	1 large	0.0	0.0	0	0
mints	14 pieces	0.6	0.0	0	0
peanut brittle	1 oz.	7.7	1.2	0	1
Peanut Butter Cups	1 oz.	9.2	3.6	3	1
Peppermint Pattie	1 oz.	3.0	2.0	0	<1
Raisinettes	1 oz.	5.5	3.0	4	0
Reese's Pieces	1.7 oz. Pkg.	13.0	5.2	2	0
sour balls	1 oz.	0.0	0.0	0	0
taffy	1 oz.	1.5	0.4	0	0
Tootsie Roll pop	1 oz.	0.6	0.2	0	0
Tootsie Roll	1 oz.	2.3	0.6	0	1

	Serving	Total Fat (g)	Sat. Fat (g)	Chol. (mg)	Fiber (g)
FATS					
bacon fat	1 T	14.0	6.4	14	0
beef, separable fat	1 oz.	23.3	6.0	24	0
butter					
solid	1 t	3.8	2.4	10	0
whipped	1 t	2.6	1.6	7	0
Butter Buds, liquid	2 T	0.0	0.0	0	0
butter sprinkles	1/2 t	0.0	0.0	0	0
chicken fat, raw	1 T	12.8	3.8	11	0
cream					
light	1 T	2.9	1.8	10	0
medium (25% fat)	1 T	3.8	2.3	13	0
whipping, light	1 T	4.6	2.9	17	0
cream substitute					
liquid/frzn	1/2 fl. oz.	1.5	1.4	0	0
powdered	1 T	0.7	0.7	0	0
half & half	1 T	1.7	1.1	6	0
margarine					
liquid or soft tub	1 t	3.8	0.6	0	0
reduced calorie tub	1 t	2.0	0.3	0	0
solid (corn), stick	1 t	3.8	0.6	0	0
fat-free tub	1 t	0.0	0.0	0	0
mayonnaise					
fat-free	1 T	0.0	0.0	0	0
reduced calorie	1 T	5.0	0.7	4	0
regular	1 T	12.0	1.3	8	0
no-stick spray (Pam, etc.)	2-sec spray	0.9	0.2	0	0
oil					
canola	1 T	13.6	1.0	0	0
corn	1 T	13.6	1.7	0	0
olive	1 T	13.5	1.8	0	0
safflower	1 T	13.6	1.2	0	0
soybean	1 T	13.6	2.0	0	0
pork fat (lard)	1 T	12.8	5.0	12	0
sandwich spread (Miracle					
Whip type)	1 T	4.9	0.7	4	0
shortening, vegetable	1 T	12.8	3.2	0	0
sour cream					
cultured	1 T	3.0	1.9	6	0
fat-free	1 T	0.0	0.0	0	0
half &half, cultured	1 T	1.8	1.1	6	0
low fat	1 T	1.8	1.1	6	0

	Serving	Total Fat (g)	Sat. Fat (g)	Chol. (mg)	Fiber (g)
FISH (all baked/broiled w/o added					
fat unless otherwise noted)					
abalone, canned	3 oz.	5.2	0.3	80	0
anchovy, canned in oil	3 fillets	1.2	0.3	10	0
bass					
freshwater	3 oz.	4.5	0.9	60	0
saltwater, black	3 oz.	1.0	0.2	50	0
saltwater, striped	3 oz.	2.3	0.6	70	0
bluefish					
cooked	3 oz.	5.2	1.3	50	0
fried	3 oz.	12.6	2.7	59	0
butterfish					
gulf	3 oz.	2.6	0.7	60	0
northern	3 oz.	10.0	1.9	49	0
carp	3 oz.	6.0	1.4	72	0
catfish	3 oz.	3.0	0.7	60	0
catfish, breaded & fried	3 oz.	13.0	2.9	75	1.0
caviar, sturgeon, granular	1 t	1.5	0.4	47	0
clams					
canned, solids & liquid	1/2 cup	0.7	0.1	25	0
meat only	5 large	1.0	0.2	42	0
soft, raw	4 large	0.8	0.1	29	0
cod					
canned	3 oz.	0.6	0.2	45	0
cooked	3 oz.	0.6	0.2	40	0
dried, salted	3 oz.	2.0	0.5	129	0
crab					
canned	1/2 cup	0.9	0.1	60	0
deviled	3 oz.	10.0	3.5	40	0
fried, cake	3 oz.	18.0	4.1	170	0
crab, Alaska king	3 oz.	1.2	0.2	53	0
crab cake	3 oz.	10.6	1.2	100	0
crayfish, freshwater	3 oz.	1.2	0.2	115	0
croaker					
Atlantic	3 oz.	3.0	1.0	60	0
white	3 oz.	0.6	0.3	60	0
dolphinfish	3 oz.	0.8	0.2	72	0
fillets, frzn					
batter dipped	2 pieces	20.0	4.0	40	1
breaded	2 pieces	18.0	3.0	35	1
fish cakes, frzn, fried	3 oz.	13.8	3.9	102	2
flounder/sole	3 oz.	0.4	0.2	30	0

	Serving	Total Fat (g)	Sat. Fat (g)	Chol. (mg)	Fiber (g)
gefilte fish	3 oz.	2.0	0.5	50	1
grouper	3 oz.	1.2	0.3	45	0
haddock					
cooked	3 oz.	0.5	0.1	50	0
fried	3 oz.	14.0	3.7	60	0
halibut	3 oz.	1.0	0.5	30	0
herring					
canned or smoked	3 oz.	16.0	6.0	66	0
cooked	3 oz.	11.0	2.0	70	0
kingfish	3 oz.	3.0	0.8	68	0
lobster					
broiled w/ butter	12 oz.	15.1	8.6	100	0
steamed	3 oz.	0.5	0.1	70	0
mackerel					
Atlantic	3 oz.	13.0	1.5	60	0
Pacific	3 oz.	12.5	1.8	55	0
mussels, meat only	3 oz.	2.0	0.7	30	0
ocean perch					
cooked	3 oz.	1.4	0.3	40	0
fried	3 oz.	11.4	2.8	62	0
octopus	3 oz.	2.0	0.4	95	0
oysters					
canned	3 oz.	2.0	0.8	54	0
fried	3 oz.	13.7	3.2	83	0
raw	5-8 medium	1.8	0.6	54	0
perch, freshwater, yellow	3 oz.	0.8	0.4	80	0
pike					
blue	3 oz.	0.7	0.5	75	0
northern	3 oz.	1.0	0.7	40	0
walleye	3 oz.	1.0	1.0	80	0
pompano	3 oz.	9.5	5.0	55	0
rainbow trout					
baked, broiled	3 oz.	5.6	1.6	70	0
breaded, fried	3 oz.	14.4	3.2	84	1
red snapper	3 oz.	1.7	0.5	35	0
rockfish, oven steamed	3 oz.	2.3	0.8	40	0
roughy, orange	3 oz.	2.0	0.1	20	0
salmon					
Atlantic	3 oz.	6.2	0.9	55	0
broiled/baked	3 oz.	7.3	2.0	50	0
chinook, canned	3 oz.	7.0	2.0	50	0
pink, canned	3 oz.	5.0	1.3	54	0

	Serving	Total Fat (g)	Sat. Fat (g)	Chol. (mg)	Fiber (g)
smoked	3 oz.	9.2	1.0	35	0
sardines					
Atlantic, in soy oil	4 sardines	7.0	0.8	67	0
skinless & boneless	3 oz.	6.0	1.5	30	0
scallops					
cooked	3 oz.	1.0	0.2	30	0
frzn, fried	3 oz.	10.3	2.3	55	0
steamed	3 oz.	1.2	0.2	40	0
sea bass, white	3 oz.	1.3	0.6	40	0
shrimp					
canned, dry pack	3 oz.	1.4	0.5	155	0
canned, wet pack	3 oz.	0.6	0.3	125	0
fried	3 oz.	10.5	0.9	120	0
raw or broiled	3 oz.	1.0	0.5	150	0
sole, fillet	3 oz.	0.3	0.2	30	0
squid					
broiled	3 oz.	1.5	0.5	250	0
fried	3 oz.	6.4	1.6	275	0
raw	3 oz.	1.2	0.4	250	0
sushi or sashimi	3 oz.	4.8	1.3	38	0
swordfish	3 oz.	4.0	1.1	43	0
trout					
brook	3 oz.	3.5	0.9	60	0
rainbow	3 oz.	7.5	1.2	85	0
tuna					
albacore	3 oz.	7.3	0.2	70	0
canned, white in oil	3 oz.	8.0	1.6	31	0
canned, white in water	3 oz.	1.5	0.5	25	0
yellowfin	3 oz.	3.0	0.5	57	0
white perch	3 oz.	3.7	0.7	65	0
whiting	3 oz.	3.0	0.4	70	0
yellowtail	3 oz.	5.2	0.9	75	0
FRUIT					
apple					
dried	1/2 cup	0.1	0.0	0	5
whole w/peel	1 medium	0.4	0.1	0	4
applesauce, unsweetened	1/2 cup	0.1	0.0	0	2
apricots					
dried	5 halves	0.2	0.0	0	6
fresh	3 medium	0.4	0.0	0	2
avocado					
California	1 (6 oz.)	30.0	4.5	0	4

	Serving	Total Fat (g)	Sat. Fat (g)	Chol. (mg)	Fiber (g)
Florida	1 (11oz.)	28.0	4.3	0	4
blackberries					
fresh	1 cup	0.6	0.0	0	7
frzn, unsweetened	1 cup	0.7	0.0	0	7
blueberries					
fresh	1 cup	0.6	0.0	0	5
frzn, unsweetened	1 cup	0.7	0.2	0	4
boysenberries, frzn unsweetened	1 cup	0.4	0.0	0	6
cantaloupe	1 cup	0.4	0.0	0	3.0
cherries	1/2 cup	0.8	0.2	0	2.0
cranberries, fresh	1 cup	0.2	0.0	0	4
cranberry sauce	1/2 cup	0.2	0.0	0	1
dates, whole, dried	1/2 cup	0.4	0.0	0	8
figs					
canned	3 figs	0.1	0.0	0	9
dried, uncooked	10 figs	1.1	0.4	0	10
fresh	1 medium	0.2	0.0	0	2
fruit cocktail, canned w/juice	1 cup	0.3	0.0	0	5
fruit roll-up	1	0.0	0.0	0	0
grapefruit	1/2 medium	0.1	0.0	0	1
grapes, seedless	1/2 cup	0.1	0.0	0	1
guava, fresh	1 medium	0.5	0.2	0	7
honeydew melon, fresh	1/4 small	0.1	0.0	0	1
kiwi, fresh	1 medium	0.3	0.0	0	2
kumquat, fresh	1 medium	0.0	0.0	0	1
lemon, fresh	1 medium	0.2	0.0	0	1
lime, fresh	1 medium	0.1	0.0	0	1
mandarin ornages, canned w/juice	1/2 cup	0.0	0.0	0	4
mango, fresh	1 medium	0.6	0.1	0	4
melon balls, frzn	1 cup	0.4	0.0	0	2
mixed fruit					
dried	1/2 cup	0.5	0.0	0	5
frzn, sweetened	1 cup	0.5	0.2	0	2
nectarine, fresh	1 medium	0.6	0.0	0	2
orange					
naval, fresh	1 medium	0.1	0.0	0	4
Valencia, fresh	1 medium	0.4	0.0	0	4
papaya, fresh	1 medium	0.4	0.1	0	3
peach					
canned, water pack	1 cup	0.1	0.0	0	4
canned in heavy syrup	1 cup	0.3	0.0	0	4
canned in light syrup	1 cup	0.1	0.0	0	4

	Serving	Total Fat (g)	Sat. Fat (g)	Chol. (mg)	Fiber (g)
fresh	1 medium	0.1	0.0	0	1
frzn, sweetened	1 cup	0.3	0.0	0	4
pear					
canned in heavy syrup	1 cup	0.3	0.0	0	6
canned in light syrup	1 cup	0.1	0.0	0	6
fresh	1 medium	0.7	0.0	0	5
persimmon, fresh	1 medium	0.1	0.0	0	3
pineapple pieces					
canned, unsweetened	1 cup	0.2	0.0	0	2
fresh	1 cup	0.7	0.0	0	3
plantain, cooked, sliced	1 cup	0.2	0.0	0	2
plum					
canned in heavy syrup	1/2 cup	0.1	0.0	0	4
fresh	1 medium	0.4	0.0	0	3
pomegranate, fresh	1 medium	0.5	0.0	0	2
prunes, dried, cooked	1/2 cup	0.2	0.0	0	10
raisins					
dark seedless	1/2 cup	0.4	0.2	0	6
golden seedless	1/2 cup	0.4	0.2	0	6
raspberries					
fresh	1 cup	0.7	0.1	0	5
frzn, sweetened	1 cup	0.4	0.0	0	10
rhubarb, stewed, unsweetened	1 cup	0.2	0.0	0	6
strawberries					
fresh	1 cup	0.6	0.0	0	3
frzn, sweetened	1 cup	0.3	0.0	0	3
frzn, unsweetened	1 cup	0.2	0.0	0	3
tangerine, fresh	1 medium	0.2	0.0	0	3
watermelon, fresh	1 cup	0.5	0.0	0	1
FRUIT JUICES					
apple juice	1 cup	0.3	0.0	0	1.0
apricot nectar	1 cup	0.2	0.0	0	2
carrot juice	1 cup	0.4	0.0	0	2
cranberry juice cocktail	1 cup	0.2	0.0	0	2
cranberry-apple juice	1 cup	0.2	0.0	0	1.5
grape juice	1 cup	0.2	0.0	0	1
grapefruit juice	1 cup	0.2	0.0	0	1.5
lemon juice	2 T	0.0	0.0	0	0
lime juice	2 T	0.0	0.0	0	0
orange juice	1 cup	0.4	0.0	0	1
peach juice or nectar	1 cup	0.1	0.0	0	1
pear juice or nectar	1 cup	0.0	0.0	0	1

	Serving	Total Fat (g)	Sat. Fat (g)	Chol. (mg)	Fiber (g)
pineapple juice	1 cup	0.2	0.0	0	1
prune juice	1 cup	0.1	0.0	0	3
tomato juice	1 cup	0.2	0.0	0	2
V8 juice	1 cup	0.1	0.0	0	2
LUNCH/DINNER COMBOS					
baked bean w/pork	1/2 cup	1.8	0.8	8	4
beans					
refried, canned	1/2 cup	1.4	0.5	5	7
refried w/fat	1/2 cup	13.2	5.2	12	7
refried, non-fat	1/2 cup	0.0	0.0	0	7
beans & franks, canned	1 cup	16.0	6.0	15	7
beef & vegetable stew	1 cup	10.5	4.9	64	2
beef goulash w/noodles	1 cup	13.9	3.6	87	2
beef noodle casserole	1 cup	19.2	6.5	81	2
beef pot pie	8 oz.	25.0	6.4	40	2
beef vegetable stew	1 cup	10.5	5.0	64	2
burrito					
bean w/cheese	1 large	11.0	5.4	26	4
bean w/o cheese	1 large	6.8	3.4	3	4
beef	1 large	19.0	10.1	70	2
cabbage roll w/beef & rice	1 medium	6.0	2.7	26	2
cannelloni, meat & cheese	1 piece	29.7	13.5	185	1
cheese souffle	1 cup	14.1	5.3	207	0
chicken a la king, hmde	1 cup	34.3	12.7	186	1
chicken a la king w/rice, frzn	1 cup	12.0	4.0	122	1
chicken & dumplings	1 cup	10.5	2.7	103	1
chicken & rice casserole	1 cup	18.0	5.1	103	1
chicken & veg. stir-fry	1 cup	6.9	1.2	26	3
chicken cacciatore, frzn	12 oz.	11.0	3.8	80	1
chicken fricassee, hmde	1 cup	18.1	5.2	85	1
chicken-fried steak	4 oz.	23.4	6.8	115	0
chicken noodle casserole	1 cup	10.7	3.2	59	2
chicken parmigiana, hmde	7 oz.	17.0	5.9	150	2
chicken pot pie	8 oz.	25.0	8.4	45	2
chicken salad, regular	1/2 cup	21.2	9.1	56	0
chicken tetrazzini	1 cup	19.6	6.9	50	1
chicken w/cashews, Chinese	1 cup	28.6	4.9	60	2
chili					
w/beans only	1 cup	12.0	4.0	35	7
w/beans & meat	1 cup	22.4	9.6	110	4
chop suey w/rice or noodles	1 cup	10.5	3.6	50	2
chow mein, chicken	1 cup	6.0	2.5	60	2

	Serving	Total Fat (g)	Sat. Fat (g)	Chol. (mg)	Fiber (g)
corned-beef hash	1 cup	24.4	7.5	80	2
crab cake	1 small	4.5	0.9	90	0
creamed chipped beef	1 cup	23.0	7.9	44	0
deviled crab	1/2 cup	15.4	4.1	50	1
deviled egg	1 large	5.3	1.2	109	0
egg foo yung w/sauce	1 piece	7.0	1.9	107	1
eggplant Parmesan, traditional	1 cup	24.0	8.7	31	3
egg roll	2	6.8	2.4	40	1
enchilada					
bean, beef & cheese	8 oz.	14.1	7.3	38	3
beef, frzn	8 oz.	16.0	8.7	40	2
cheese, frzn	8 oz.	26.3	14.7	61	3
chicken, frzn	8 oz.	16.1	6.4	65	4
fajitas					
chicken	1	15.3	3.0	41	4
beef	1	18.2	6.1	34	3
fettuccine Alfredo	1 cup	29.7	9.3	73	3
fish and chips, frzn dinner	6 oz.	14.8	4.3	25	3
fish creole	1 cup	5.4	0.9	60	2
frzn dinner					
beef tips and noodles	12 oz.	15.1	6.2	75	4
chopped sirloin	12 oz.	30.1	14.3	130	5
fried chicken	12 oz.	29.6	7.4	110	6
meat loaf	12 oz.	23.1	6.4	65	4
Salisbury steak	12 oz.	27.4	13.5	126	4
turkey and dressing	12 oz.	22.6	5.0	74	3
green pepper stuffed w/rice & beef	1 medium	13.5	5.8	52	2
hamburger rice casserole	1 cup	21.0	7.7	57	3
ham salad w/mayo	1/2 cup	20.2	4.4	54	0
lasagna					
cheese	8 oz.	12.0	4.8	22	3
w/beef & cheese	1 piece	19.8	10.0	81	2
lobster					
Cantonese	1 cup	19.6	5.6	240	0
Newburg	1/2 cup	24.8	14.7	183	0
salad	1/2 cup	7.0	1.5	36	0
lo mein, Chinese	1 cup	7.2	1.4	11	1
macaroni & cheese	1 cup	16.0	5.0	20	0
manicotti, cheese & tomato	1 piece	11.8	6.0	61	2
meatball (reg. ground beef)	1 medium	5.1	2.0	30	0
meat loaf w/reg. ground beef	3 oz.	20.2	8.5	102	0
moo goo gai pan	1 cup	17.2	3.1	66	1

	Serving	Total Fat (g)	Sat. Fat (g)	Chol. (mg)	Fiber (g)
moussaka	1 cup	8.9	2.8	98	3
onion rings	10 average	17.0	6.0	0	1
oysters Rockefeller	6 oysters	12.5	4.0	70	1
pepper steak	1 cup	11.0	3.2	53	1
pizza					
cheese	1 slice	10.1	5.2	40	1
cheese, French bread, frzn	5 oz.	13.0	6.7	37	1
combination w/meat	1 slice	17.5	9.0	56	1
deep dish, cheese	1 slice	13.5	6.9	45	1
pepperoni	1 slice	16.5	8.5	44	1
tomato only	1 slice	4.0	2.0	2	1
pizza rolls, frzn	3 pieces	6.9	2.0	10	1
pork, sweet & sour w/rice	1 cup	7.5	2.0	31	1
quiche					
Lorraine	1/8 pie	43.5	20.1	218	1
plain or vegetable	1 slice	17.6	8.8	135	1
ratatouille	1/2 cup	3.0	0.7	0	2
ravioli, canned	1 cup	7.3	3.6	20	3
ravioli w/meat & tomato sauce	1 piece	3.0	0.9	19	0
Salisbury steak w/gravy	8 oz.	27.3	12.3	126	1
salmon patty, traditional	4 oz.	12.5	4.1	94	1
sandwiches (on whole wheat bread					
unless otherwise noted)					
BBQ beef on bun	1	16.8	5.8	54	4
BBQ pork on bun	1	12.2	3.7	56	4
BLT w/mayo	1	15.6	4.1	23	4
bologna & cheese	1	22.5	9.7	42	4
chicken w/mayo & lettuce	1	14.2	1.8	119	4
club w/mayo	1	20.8	5.4	52	4
corned beef on rye	1	10.8	3.2	34	4
cream cheese & jelly	1	16.0	10.8	38	4
egg salad	1	12.5	2.5	228	4
french dip, au jus	1	12.5	4.8	58	4
grilled cheese	1	24.0	12.4	56	4
ham, cheese & mayo	1	16.0	7.3	29	4
ham salad w/mayo	1	16.9	4.2	40	4
peanut butter & jelly	1	15.1	2.3	10	5
Reuben	1	33.3	11.8	77	4
roast beef & gravy	1	24.5	5.6	55	4
roast beef & mayo	1	22.6	4.9	60	4
sloppy joe on bun	1	16.8	5.8	54	4
sub w/salami & cheese	1	41.3	17.7	109	4

	Serving	Total Fat (g)	Sat. Fat (g)	Chol. (mg)	Fiber (g)
tuna salad	1	17.5	2.9	17	4
turkey & mayo	1	18.4	1.9	17	4
turkey breast & mustard	1	5.2	1.2	15	4
shrimp creole w/rice	1 cup	6.1	1.2	123	2
shrimp salad	1/2 cup	9.5	1.6	69	1
spaghetti					
w/marinara sauce	1 cup	2.5	1.0	5	2
w/meat sauce	1 cup	16.7	5.0	56	2
w/red clam sauce	1 cup	7.3	1.0	17	2
w/tomato sauce	1 cup	1.5	0.4	5	2
w/white clam sauce	1 cup	19.5	2.6	49	1
SpaghettiOs	1 cup	2.0	0.5	8	2
spinach souffle	1 cup	14.8	7.1	184	2
stroganoff					
beef w/noodles	1 cup	19.6	7.7	72	2
beef w/o noodles	1 cup	26.8	10.6	85	1
sushi w/fish & vegetables	5 oz.	1.0	0.2	10	1
taco, beef	1 medium	17.0	8.5	54	2
tortellini, meat or cheese	1 cup	15.4	5.4	238	1
tostada w/refried beans	1 medium	16.3	6.7	20	6
tuna noodle casserole	1 cup	13.3	3.1	38	2
tuna salad					
oil pack w/mayo	1/2 cup	16.3	2.7	20	0
water pack w/mayo	1/2 cup	10.5	1.6	14	0
veal parmigiana	1 cup	22.5	10.1	75	0
veal scallopini	1 cup	20.4	7.3	132	2
Welsh rarebit	1 cup	31.6	17.3	NA	0
MEATS (all cooked w/o added fat unless otherwise noted					
round, eye of, lean	3 oz.	4.0	1.5	52	0
beef, lean, 5-10% fat by weight (cooked)					
flank steak, fat trimmed	3 oz.	8.0	2.9	82	0
hindshank, lean	3 oz.	9.2	4.0	76	0
porterhouse steak, lean	3 oz.	10.2	5.3	90	0
rib steak, lean	3 oz.	9.2	5.0	80	0
round bottom, lean	3 oz.	9.2	3.4	96	0
roasted	3 oz.	7.2	2.7	81	0
rump, lean, pot-roasted	3 oz.	7.0	2.5	60	0
top, lean	3 oz.	6.2	2.2	89	0
sirloin steak, lean	3 oz.	8.7	3.6	76	0
sirloin tip, lean roasted	3 oz.	9.2	3.9	90	0
tenderloin, lean, broiled	3 oz.	11.0	4.2	83	0
top sirloin, lean, broiled	3 oz.	7.7	3.1	89	0

	Serving	Total Fat (g)	Sat. Fat (g)	Chol. (mg)	Fiber (g)
beef, regular, 11-17.4% fat by weight (cooked)					
chuck, separable lean	3 oz.	15.0	6.2	105	0
club steak, lean	3 oz.	12.7	6.1	90	0
cubed steak	3 oz.	15.2	3.3	85	0
hamburger					
extra lean	3 oz.	13.9	6.3	82	0
lean	3 oz.	15.7	7.2	78	0
rib roast, lean	3 oz.	15.0	5.5	85	0
sirloin tips, roasted	3 oz.	15.0	3.2	85	0
T-bone, lean only	4 oz.	10.2	4.2	80	0
terderloin, marbled	3 oz.	15.0	7.0	86	0
beef, high fat, 17.4-27.4% fat by weight (cooked)					
chuck, ground	3 oz.	23.7	9.6	100	0
hamburger, regular	3 oz.	19.6	8.2	87	0
meatballs	1 oz.	5.5	2.0	30	0
porterhouse steak, lean &					
marbled	3 oz.	19.5	8.2	80	0
rib steak	3 oz.	14.5	6.0	81	0
rump, pot-roasted	3 oz.	19.5	8.2	80	0
short ribs, lean	3 oz.	19.5	8.2	80	0
sirloin, broiled	3 oz.	18.5	7.7	78	0
sirloin, ground	3 oz.	26.5	9.3	84	0
T-bone, broiled	3 oz.	26.5	10.5	90	0
beef, highest fat, =27.5% fat by weight (cooked)					
brisket, lean & marbled	3 oz.	30.0	12.0	85	0
chuck, stew meat	3 oz.	30.0	12.0	85	0
corned, medium fat	3 oz.	30.0	14.9	75	0
ribeye steak, marbled	3 oz.	38.6	12.0	90	0
rib roast	3 oz.	30.0	18.2	85	0
short ribs	3 oz.	31.5	10.5	90	0
lamb					
leg					
lean	3 oz.	8.0	3.4	100	0
lean & marbled	3 oz.	14.3	9.0	97	0
loin chop					
lean	3 oz.	8.0	4.2	80	0
lean & marbled	3 oz.	22.3	11.7	58	0
rib chop					
lean	3 oz.	8.0	5.0	50	0
lean & marbled	3 oz.	21.0	13.0	70	0
liver					
beef, braised	3 oz.	4.8	1.9	400	0

	Serving	Total Fat (g)	Sat. Fat (g)	Chol. (mg)	Fiber (g)
calf, braised	3 oz.	6.8	2.3	450	0
pork					
bacon					
cured, broiled	1 strip	3.1	1.1	5	0
cured, raw	1 oz.	16.3	6.0	19	0
Canadian bacon, broiled	1 oz.	1.8	0.6	14	0
ham					
cured, canned	3 oz.	5.0	1.5	38	0
cured, shank, lean	3 oz.	6.2	3.0	59	0
marbled	2 slices	13.8	5.0	60	0
fresh, lean	3 oz.	6.3	1.5	40	0
smoked	3 oz.	7.0	2.7	51	0
smoked, 95% lean	3 oz.	5.3	1.8	53	0
loin chop					
lean	1 chop	7.7	3.0	55	0
lean with fat	1 chop	22.5	8.8	90	0
rib chop, trimmed	3 oz.	9.8	3.5	81	0
rib roast, trimmed	3 oz.	10.0	3.6	83	0
sausage					
brown and serve	1 oz.	9.4	3.1	24	0
patty	1	8.4	2.9	22	0
regular link	1/2 oz.	4.7	1.6	15	0
sirloin, lean, roasted	3 oz.	10.0	3.6	85	0
spareribs roasted	6 medium	35.0	11.8	121	0
tenderloin, lean, roast	3 oz.	4.6	1.6	78	0
top loin roast, trimmed	3 oz.	7.5	2.8	77	0
processed meats					
bacon substitute (breakfast					
strips)	2 strips	4.8	1.0	0	0
beef, chipped	2 slices	1.1	0.4	15	0
beef breakfast strips	2 strips	7.0	2.8	26	0
beef jerky	1 oz.	3.6	1.7	30	0
bologna, beef/beef & pork	2 oz.	16.2	6.9	33	0
bratwurst					
pork	2 oz. link	22.0	7.9	51	0
pork & beef	2 oz. link	19.5	7.0	44	0
chicken roll	2 oz.	2.6	1.6	20	0
corn dog	1	20.0	8.4	37	0
corned beef, jellied	1 oz.	2.9	1.0	3	0
ham, chopped	1 oz.	2.3	0.8	17	0
hot dog/frank					
beef	1	13.2	8.8	27	0

	Serving	Total Fat (g)	Sat. Fat (g)	Chol. (mg)	Fiber (g)
beef, fat-free	1	0.0	0.0	0	0
chicken	1	8.8	2.5	45	0
97% fat-free varieties	1	1.6	0.6	22	0
turkey	1	8.1	2.7	39	0
turkey, fat-free	1	0.0	0.0	0	0
knockwurst/knackwurst	2 oz. link	18.9	3.2	36	0
pepperoni	1 oz.	13.0	5.4	25	0
salami					
cooked	1 oz.	10.0	6.6	30	0
dry/hard	1 oz.	10.0	3.0	16	0
sausage					
Italian	2 oz. link	17.2	6.1	52	0
90% fat-free varieties	2 oz.	4.6	1.6	40	0
Polish	2 oz. link	16.2	5.8	40	0
smoked	2 oz. link	20.0	9.2	48	0
Vienna	1 sausage	4.0	1.5	8	0
turkey breast, smoked	2 oz.	1.0	0.3	23	0
turkey ham	2 oz.	2.9	1.0	32	0
turkey loaf	2 oz.	1.0	0.3	23	0
turkey roll, light meat	2 oz.	4.1	1.2	24	0
veal					
blade					
lean	3 oz.	8.3	3.5	100	0
lean with fat	3 oz.	16.5	7.0	100	0
breast, stewed	3 oz.	18.5	8.7	100	0
chuck, med. fat, brasied	3 oz.	12.6	6.0	101	0
cutlet breaded	3 1/2 oz.	15.0	NA	NA	0
NUTS AND SEEDS					
almonds	2 T	9.3	1.0	0	2.5
Brazil nuts	2 T	11.5	2.3	0	2.5
cashews, roasted	2 T	7.8	1.3	0	2
chestnuts, fresh	2 T	0.8	0.0	0	4
hazelnuts (filberts)	2 T	10.6	1.0	0	2
macadamia nuts, roasted	2 T	12.3	2.0	0	2.5
mixed nuts					
w/peanuts	2 T	10.0	1.5	0	2
w/o peanuts	2 T	10.1	2.0	0	2
peanut butter, creamy	1 T	8.0	1.5	0	1
peanut butter, chunky		8.5	2.5	0	2
peanuts					
chopped	2 T	8.9	1.0	0	2
honey roasted	2 T	8.9	1.5	0	2

	Serving	Total Fat (g)	Sat. Fat (g)	Chol. (mg)	Fiber (g)
in shell	1 cup	17.0	2.2	0	4
pecans	2 T	9.1	0.5	0	1
pine nuts (pignolia)	2 T	9.1	1.5	0	2
pistachios	2 T	7.7	0.8	0	2
poppy seeds	1 T	3.8	0.3	0	2
pumpkin seeds	2 T	7.9	3.0	0	2
sesame nut mix	2 T	5.1	1.5	0	2
sesame seeds	2 T	8.8	1.2	0	2
sunflower seeds	2 T	8.9	1.0	0	2
trail mix w/seeds, nuts, carob	2 T	5.1	0.9	0	3
walnuts	2 T	7.7	0.3	0	2.5
PASTA, NOODLES AND RICE					
macaroni					
semolina	1 cup	0.7	0.0	0	1
whole wheat	1 cup	2.0	0.4	0	3.5
noodles					
Alfredo	1 cup	25.1	9.8	73	1
Angel Hair	1 cup	1.5	0.5	0	0
cellophone, fried	1 cup	4.2	0.6	0	0
chow mein	1 cup	8.0	1.6	0	0
egg	1 cup	2.4	0.4	50	1
fettuccine, spinach	1 cup	2.0	0.5	0	2
manicotti	1 cup	1.0	0.2	0	1
ramen, all varieties	1 cup	8.0	5.0	0	1
rice	1 cup	0.3	0.0	0	1
romanoff	1 cup	18.0	11.9	95	3
spaghetti, whole wheat	1 cup	1.5	0.5	0	3
spaghetti, enriched	1 cup	1.0	0.0	0	1
rice					2
brown	1/2 cup	0.6	0.0	0	1
fried	1/2 cup	7.2	0.7	0	2
long grain & wild	1/2 cup	2.1	0.2	0	1
pilaf	1/2 cup	7.0	0.6	0	1
Spanish style	1/2 cup	2.1	1.0	0	0
white	1/2 cup	1.2	0.0	0	0
POULTRY					
chicken					
breast					
w/skin, fried	1/2 breast	10.7	3.0	87	0
w/o skin, fried	1/2 breast	6.1	1.5	90	0
w/skin, roasted	1/2 breast	7.6	2.9	70	0
w/o skin, roasted	1/2 breast	3.1	1.0	80	0

	Serving	Total Fat (g)	Sat. Fat (g)	Chol. (mg)	Fiber (g)
leg					
w/skin, fried	1 leg	8.7	4.4	99	0
w/skin, roasted	1 leg	4.8	4.2	85	0
w/o skin, roasted	1 leg	2.5	0.7	41	0
thigh					
w/skin, fried	1 thigh	11.3	2.5	60	0
w/skin, roasted	1 thigh	9.6	2.7	58	0
w/o skin, roasted	1 thigh	4.5	2.4	45	0
wing					
w/skin, fried	1 wing	9.1	1.9	26	0
w/skin, roasted	1 wing	6.6	1.9	29	0
duck					
w/skin, roasted	3 oz.	28.7	9.7	84	0
w/o skin, roasted	3 oz.	11.0	4.2	89	0
turkey breast					
barbecued	3 oz.	3.0	1.3	42	0
honey roasted	3 oz.	2.6	1.1	38	0
oven roasted	3 oz.	3.0	1.3	42	0
smoked	3 oz.	3.3	1.4	49	0
dark meat					
w/skin, roasted	3 oz.	11.3	3.5	89	0
w/o skin, roasted	3 oz.	7.0	2.4	75	0
ground	3 oz.	13.2	4.0	85	0
ham	3 oz.	5.0	1.7	62	0
light meat					
w/skin, roasted	3 oz.	8.2	2.3	76	0
w/o skin, roasted	3 oz.	3.2	1.0	55	0
roll, light meat	3 oz.	7.0	2.0	43	0
sliced w/gravy, frzn	3 oz.	3.7	1.2	20	0
SALAD DRESSINGS					
blue cheese					
fat free	1 T	0.0	0.0	0	0
low cal	1 T	1.9	0.2	2	0
regular	1 T	8.0	1.4	0	0
buttermilk, from mix	1 T	5.8	1.0	5	0
Caesar	1 T	7.0	0.9	13	0
French					
fat free	1 T	0.0	0.0	0	0
low cal	1 T	0.9	0.1	1	0
regular	1 T	6.4	0.8	0	0
garlic, from mix	1 T	9.2	1.4	0	0
honey mustard	1 T	6.6	1.0	0	0

	Serving	Total Fat (g)	Sat. Fat (g)	Chol. (mg)	Fiber (g)
Italian					
creamy	1 T	5.5	1.6	0	0
fat free	1 T	0.0	0.0	0	0
low cal	1 T	1.5	0.1	1	0
oil & vinegar	1 T	7.5	1.5	0	0
ranch style	1 T	6.0	0.8	4	0
Russian					
low cal	1 T	0.7	0.1	1	0
regular	1 T	7.8	1.1	0	0
Thousand Island					
fat free	1 T	0.0	0.0	0	0
low cal	1 T	1.6	0.2	2	0
regular	1 T	5.6	0.9	0	0
SAUCES AND GRAVIES					
barbecue sauce	1 T	0.3	0.0	0	0
bearnaise sauce, mix	1/4 cup	25.6	15.7	71	0
beef gravy, canned	1/2 cup	2.8	1.3	4	0
brown gravy					
from mix	1/2 cup	0.9	0.4	1	0
hmde	1/4 cup	14.0	6.5	5	0
catsup, tomato	1 T	0.1	0.0	0	0
chicken gravy					
canned	1/2 cup	6.8	1.7	3	0
from mix	1/2 cup	0.9	0.3	1	0
giblet, hmde	1/4 cup	2.6	0.7	28	0
chili sauce	1 T	0.0	0.0	0	0
cocktail sauce	1/4 cup	0.2	0.0	0	0
guacamole dip	1 oz.	4.0	0.7	0	0
hollandaise sauce	1/4 cup	18.0	10.2	160	0
home-style gravy, from mix	1/4 cup	0.5	0.2	0	0
horseradish	1/4 cup	0.1	0.0	0	0
jalapeno dip	1 oz.	1.1	0.4	60	0
mushroom gravy					
canned	1/2 cup	3.2	0.5	0	1
from mix	1/2 cup	0.4	0.2	0	1
mustard					
brown	1 T	1.8	0.3	0	1
yellow	1 T	0.7	0.0	0	0
onion dip	2 T	6.0	3.7	13	0
onion gravy, from mix	1/2 cup	0.4	0.2	0	0
pesto sauce	1/4 cup	29.0	7.3	18	1
picante sauce	1/2 cup	0.8	0.1	0	2

	Serving	Total Fat (g)	Sat. Fat (g)	Chol. (mg)	Fiber (g)
pork gravy, from mix	1/2 cup	1.0	0.4	1	0
sour-cream sauce	1/4 cup	7.6	4.0	28	0
soy sauce	1 T	0.0	0.0	0	0
soy sauce, reduced sodium	1 T	0.0	0.0	0	0
spaghetti sauce					
"healthy"/"lite" varieties	1/2 cup	1.0	0.0	0	3
hmde, w/ground beef	1/2 cup	8.3	2.3	23	2
marinara	1/2 cup	4.7	0.7	0	3
meat flavor, jar	1/2 cup	6.0	1.0	5	2
mushroom, jar	1/2 cup	2.0	0.3	0	2
oil & garlic	1/2 cup	4.5	1.5	5	0
tomato	1/2 cup	2.2	0.5	0	0
spinach dip (sour-cream & mayo)	2 T	7.1	1.8	10	1
steak sauce					
A-1	1 T	0.0	0.0	0	0
others	1 T	0.0	0.0	0	0
tabasco sauce	1 t	0.0	0.0	0	0
tartar sauce	1 T	8.2	1.5	0	0
teriyaki sauce	1 T	0.0	0.0	0	0
turkey gravy					
canned	1/2 cup	2.4	0.7	3	0
from mix	1/2 cup	0.9	0.3	1	0
Worcestershire sauce	1 T	0.0	0.0	0	0
SOUPS					
asparagus					
cream of, w/milk	1 cup	8.2	2.1	10	1
cream of, w/water	1 cup	4.1	1.0	5	1
bean					
w/bacon	1 cup	5.9	6.0	3	4
w/ham	1 cup	8.5	2.0	3	3
w/o meat	1 cup	3.0	1.5	2	5
beef					
broth	1 cup	0.5	0.2	1	0
chunky	1 cup	5.1	2.6	14	2
beef barley	1 cup	1.1	0.5	6	1
beef noodle	1 cup	3.1	1.2	5	1
black bean	1 cup	1.5	1.2	0	2
broccoli, creamy w/water	1 cup	2.8	1.0	5	1
canned vegetable type w/o meat	1 cup	1.6	0.6	0	1
chicken					
chunky	1 cup	6.6	2.0	30	2
cream of, w/milk	1 cup	11.5	4.6	27	0

	Serving	Total Fat (g)	Sat. Fat (g)	Chol. (mg)	Fiber (g)
cream of, w/water	1 cup	7.4	2.1	10	0
chicken & dumplings	1 cup	5.5	1.3	34	0
chicken & stars	1 cup	1.8	0.7	5	1
chicken & wild rice	1 cup	2.3	0.5	7	1
chicken/beef noodle or veg.	1 cup	3.1	1.2	5	1
chicken gumbo	1 cup	1.4	0.3	5	1
chicken mushroom	1 cup	9.2	2.4	10	1
chicken noodle					
chunky	1 cup	5.2	1.1	18	2
w/water	1 cup	2.5	0.7	7	0
chicken vegetable					
chunky	1 cup	4.8	1.4	17	2
w/water	1 cup	2.8	0.9	10	0
chicken w/noodles, chunky	1 cup	5.0	1.4	19	2
chicken w/rice					
chunky	1 cup	3.2	1.0	20	2
w/water	1 cup	1.9	0.5	7	1
clam chowder					
Manhattan chunky	1 cup	3.4	2.1	14	1
New England	1 cup	6.6	3.6	7	1
consomme w/gelatin	1 cup	0.0	0.0	0	0
corn chowder	1 cup	10.5	5.0	22	3.5
crab	1 cup	1.5	0.4	10	0
fish chowder, w/whole milk	1 cup	13.5	5.3	37	1
gazpacho	1 cup	1.5	0.5	0	3
seafood gumbo	1 cup	3.9	2.7	40	3
lentil	1 cup	1.0	0.2	0	3
lobster bisque	1 cup	14.0	5.5	35	1
minestrone					
chunky	1 cup	2.8	1.5	5	2
w/water	1 cup	2.5	0.8	3	1
mushroom, cream of					
condensed	1 cup	23.1	10.1	30	1
w/milk	1 cup	13.6	5.1	20	1
w/water	1 cup	9.0	2.4	2	1
mushroom barley	1 cup	2.3	0.4	0	1
mushroom w/beef stock	1 cup	4.0	1.6	7	1
onion	1 cup	1.7	0.3	0	1
onion, French w/cheese	1 cup	7.5	2.5	15	0
oyster stew w/water	1 cup	3.8	2.5	14	1
oyster stew w/whole milk	1 cup	17.7	2.5	14	0
pea					

	Serving	Total Fat (g)	Sat. Fat (g)	Chol. (mg)	Fiber (g)
split	1 cup	0.6	0.2	1	1
split w/ham	1 cup	4.4	1.8	8	1
potato, cream of w/milk-	1 cup	7.4	1.2	5	2
tomato					
w/milk	1 cup	6.0	2.9	17	1
w/water	1 cup	1.9	0.4	0	0.5
tomato beef w/noodle	1 cup	4.3	1.6	5	1
tomato rice	1 cup	2.7	0.5	2	1
turkey noodle	1 cup	2.0	0.6	5	1
turkey vegetable	1 cup	3.0	0.9	2	1
vegetable, chunky	1 cup	3.7	0.6	0	2
vegetable w/beef, chunky	1 cup	3.0	1.3	8	2
vegetable w/beef broth	1 cup	1.9	0.4	2	1
vegetarian vegetable	1 cup	1.2	0.3	0	1
wonton	1 cup	1.0	<1.0	10	1
VEGETABLES					
alfalfa sprouts, raw	1/2 cup	0.1	0.0	0	0
artichoke, boiled	1 medium	0.2	0.0	0	3
atichoke hearts, boiled	1/2 cup	0.1	0.0	0	3
asparagus, cooked	1/2 cup	0.3	0.1	0	2
avocado	1/2 cup	25.0	4.0	0	3.5
bamboo shoots, raw	1/2 cup	0.2	0.1	0	2
beans					
all types, cooked w/o fat	1/2 cup	0.4	0.2	0	9
baked, brown sugar &					
molasses	1/2 cup	1.5	0.2	0	4
baked, vegetarian	1/2 cup	0.6	0.3	0	5
baked w/pork & tomato					
sauce	1/2 cup	1.3	0.5	8	5
beets, pickled	1/2 cup	0.1	0.0	0	4
broccoli					
cooked	1/2 cup	0.3	0.0	0	7
frzn, chopped, cooked	1/2 cup	0.1	0.0	0	2
frzn in butter sauce	1/2 cup	1.5	1.0	<5	2
raw	1/2 cup	0.2	0.0	0	1
brussel sprouts, cooked	1/2 cup	0.4	0.0	0	2
butter beans, canned	1/2 cup	0.4	0.0	0	4
cabbage					
Chinese (Bok Choy)	1 cup	0.2	0.0	0	2
green, cooked	1/2 cup	0.1	0.0	0	2
carrot					
cooked	1/2 cup	0.1	0.0	0	2

	Serving	Total Fat (g)	Sat. Fat (g)	Chol. (mg)	Fiber (g)
raw	1 large	0.1	0.0	0	2
cauliflower					
cooked	1 cup	0.2	0.0	0	3
raw	1 cup	0.1	0.0	0	4
celery					
cooked	1/2 cup	0.1	0.0	0	1
raw	1 stalk	0.1	0.0	0	1
Chinese-style vegetables, frzn	1/2 cup	4.0	0.2	0	3
chives, raw, chopped	1 T	0.0	0.0	0	0
collard green, cooked	1/2 cup	0.1	0.0	0	2
corn					
corn on the cob	1 medium	1.0	0.1	0	4
cream style, canned	1/2 cup	0.5	0.1	0	4
frzn, cooked	1/2 cup	0.1	0.0	0	4
cucumber					
w/skin	1/2 medium	0.2	0.0	0	1
w/o skin, sliced	1/2 cup	0.1	0.0	0	0
eggplant, cooked	1/2 cup	0.1	0.0	0	2
green beans					
french style, cooked	1/2 cup	0.2	0.0	0	2
snap, cooked	1/2 cup	0.2	0.0	0	2
Italian-style vegetables, frzn	1/2 cup	5.5	0.2	0	2
kale, cooked	1/2 cup	0.3	0.0	0	2
kidney beans, red, cooked	1/2 cup	0.5	0.0	0	8
leeks, chopped, raw	1/4 cup	0.1	0.0	0	1
lentils, cooked	1/2 cup	0.4	0.0	0	8
lettuce, leaf	1 cup	0.2	0.0	0	1
lima beans, cooked	1/2 cup	0.4	0.0	0	5
mushrooms					
canned	1/2 cup	0.2	0.0	0	1
raw	1/2 cup	0.2	0.0	0	1
mustard greens, cooked	1/2 cup	0.2	0.0	0	2
okra, cooked	1/2 cup	0.1	0.0	0	3
olives					
black	3 med	4.5	0.5	0	1
greek	3 med	5.0	0.9	0	1
green	3 med	2.5	0.2	0	1
onions					
canned, french fried	1 oz.	15.0	6.9	0	0
chopped, raw	1/2 cup	0.1	0.0	0	1
parsley, chopped, raw	1/4 cup	0.1	0.0	0	0
peas, green, cooked	1/2 cup	0.2	0.0	0	4

	Serving	Total Fat (g)	Sat. Fat (g)	Chol. (mg)	Fiber (g)
pickles	1 medium	0.1	0.0	0	0
pepper, bell, chopped, raw	1/2 cup	0.1	0.0	0	2
pimentos, canned	1 oz.	0.0	0.0	0	0
potato					
baked w/skin	1 medium	0.2	0.1	0	4
boiled w/o skin	1/2 cup	0.1	0.0	0	2
french fries	1/2 cup	6.8	3.0	10	2
hash browns	1/2 cup	10.9	3.4	23	2
mashed w/milk	1/2 cup	5.0	1.5	5	1
potato panckes	1 cake	12.6	3.4	93	1
scalloped	1/2 cup	6.0	3.5	12	1
pumpkin, canned	1/2 cup	0.3	0.2	0	4
radish, raw	1/2 cup	0.2	0.0	0	1
rhubarb, raw	1 cup	0.2	0.0	0	2
sauerkraut, canned	1/2 cup	0.2	0.0	0	4
scallions, raw	1/2 cup	0.2	0.0	0	4
soybeans, mature, cooked	1/2 cup	7.7	1.1	0	4
spinach					
cooked	1/2 cup	0.2	0.1	0	3
creamed	1/2 cup	5.1	0.7	1	3
raw	1 cup	0.2	0.0	0	3
squash	1/2 cup	0.2	0.0	0	3
succotash, cooked	1/2 cup	0.8	0.1	0	3
sweet potato					
baked	1 medium	0.2	0.0	0	6
candied	1/2 cup	3.4	1.2	8	5
tempeh (soybean product)	1/2 cup	6.4	0.9	0	1
tofu (soybean curd), raw	1/2 cup	5.4	0.8	0	1
tomato					
boiled	1/2 cup	0.5	0.0	0	1
raw	1 medium	0.4	0.0	0	1
stewed	1/2 cup	0.2	0.0	0	1
turnip greens, cooked	1/2 cup	0.2	0.0	0	2
wax beans, canned	1/2 cup	0.2	0.0	0	2
yam, boiled/baked	1/2 cup	0.1	0.0	0	3
zucchini, cooked	1/2 cup	0.1	0.0	0	2
VARIOUS SNACKS					
cheese puffs	1 oz.	10.0	4.8	14	0
cheese straws	4 pieces	7.2	6.4	5	1
Chex snack mix, traditional	1 oz.	4.0	0.5	0	1
corn chips					
barbecue	1 oz.	9.0	0.2	0	1

	Serving	Total Fat (g)	Sat. Fat (g)	Chol. (mg)	Fiber (g)
regular	1 oz.	10.0	1.0	0	1
Cracker Jack	1 oz.	2.2	0.3	0	2
mix (cereal & pretzels)	1 cup	2.5	0.5	0	2
mix (raisins & nuts)	1 cup	25.0	3.5	1.5	4.0
peanuts in shell	1 cup	17.0	2.2	0	4
popcorn					
air popped	1 cup	0.3	0.0	0	1
caramel	1 cup	4.5	1.2	2	1
mircowave, "lite"	1 cup	1.0	0.0	0	1
microwave, plain	1 cup	3.0	0.7	0	1
microwave, w/butter	1 cup	4.5	1.8	1	1
pork rinds	1 oz.	9.3	3.7	24	0
potato chips					
regular	1 oz.	11.2	2.9	0	1
baked, Lays	1 oz.	1.5	0.0	0	2
barbecue favor	1 oz.	9.5	2.6	0	1
light, Pringles	1 oz.	8.0	2.0	0	0
regular, Pringles	1 oz.	12.0	2.0	0	0
pretzels (hard)	1 oz.	1.5	0.5	0	1
Supcrpretzel® (soft)	1 med.	1.0	0.0	0	2
rice cakes	1	0.0	0.0	0	0
tortilla chips					
Doritos	1 oz.	6.6	1.1	0	1
no oil, baked	1 oz.	1.5	1.0	0	1
Tostitos	1 oz.	7.8	1.1	0	1

STEP 2:
FIT-STEP®

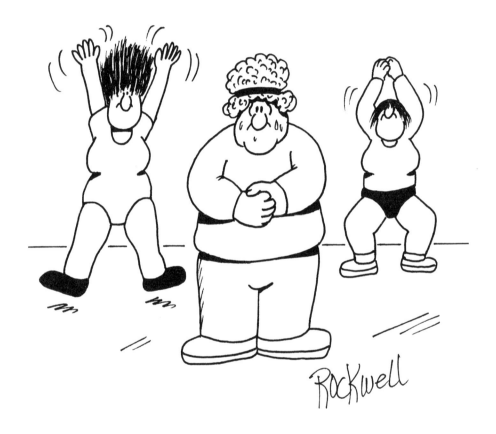

"MY PULSE RATE HAS REACHED ITS TARGET GOAL. IF THAT'S SUPPOSED TO BE SO GOOD FOR ME, THEN WHY DO I FEEL SO BAD?"

CHAPTER 7

ONLY 20 MINUTES FOR AEROBIC FITNESS

****

TAKE THAT FIRST STEP FOR ENERGY, FITNESS AND PEP

With the advent of the computer age, women are forced by design to do less and less physical labor. It would seem logical that this would result in more energy being available for other activities. However, how many times have you noticed that the less you do, the more tired you feel, whereas the more active you are, the more energy you have for other activities? Exercise improves the efficiency of the lungs, the heart and the circulatory system in their ability to take in and deliver *oxygen* throughout the entire body. This *oxygen* is the catalyst which burns the fuel (food) we take in to produce energy. Consequently, the more oxygen we take in, the more *energy* we have for all of our activities.

Oxygen is the vital ingredient which is necessary for our survival. Since oxygen can't be stored, our cells need a continuous supply in order to remain healthy. Walking increases your body's ability to extract oxygen from the air, so that increased amounts of oxygen are available for every organ, tissue and cell in the body. Walking actually increases the *total volume* of blood, making more red blood cells available to carry oxygen and nutrition to the tissues, and to remove carbon dioxide and waste products from the body's cells. This increased saturation of the tissues with oxygen is also aided by the opening of *small blood vessels,* which is another direct result of walking.

So let's take that first step for energy, fitness and pep. Walking every day will keep a fresh supply of oxygen surging through your blood vessels to all of your body's hungry cells. Don't disappoint these little fellows because you depend on them as much as they depend on you. If you short-change them on their daily oxygen supply, they'll take it out on you in the form of illness and disease. *A Fit-Step® a day keeps the doctor away.*

20 MINUTES POWERS THE DIET-STEP® DIET

<u>Twenty minutes</u> everyday except Sunday is all that you need to complete the <u>FIT-STEP® PLAN.</u> Either 20 minutes outdoors (walking) or 20 minutes indoors (stationary bike or treadmill) will provide you with maximum cardiovascular fitness, good health, and boundless energy. Remember, this 20 minute walk is a basic part of your weight loss program in the <u>Diet-Step®</u> diet. The 20 minute walk 6 days per week is what burns the extra calories needed to lose weight and to decrease your appetite when you're on the <u>Diet-Step®</u> diet. The Fit-Step® walking plan also provides the fuel that powers your energy level throughout your day.

ON YOUR MARK, GET SET, DO THE FIT-STEP®

When you first start your Fit-step® walking program, pick a level terrain, since hills place too much strain and stress on your legs, hips and back muscles. Concentrate on maintaining *erect posture* while walking. Walk with your shoulders relaxed and your arms carried in a relatively low position with natural motion at the elbow. Don't hold your arms too high when you walk, otherwise you will develop muscle spasms and pain in your neck, back and shoulder muscles.

Make sure you walk at a *brisk pace* (approximately 3 to 3 ½ mph) for maximum efficiency. When you begin walking, your respiration and heart rate will automatically become faster; however, if you feel short of breath or tired, then you're probably walking too fast. Remember to stop whenever you are tired or fatigued and then resume walking after resting. Concentrate on walking naturally, putting *energy* into each step. Soon you will begin to feel relaxed and comfortable as your stride becomes smooth and effortless. Walk with an even *steady* gait and your own rhythm of walking will automatically develop into an unconscious synchronous movement.

ONLY 4 WEEKS TO REACH YOUR PEAK

Your Fit-Step® walking program should be planned to meet your individual schedule; however, when you begin it's a good idea to walk at a specific time every day to ensure regularity and consistency. You will be able to vary your schedule once you have started the program. Lunchtime, for example, is an ideal time to plan a 20 minute walk since it combines both calorie burning and calorie reduction. If you have less time for lunch, you'll eat less.

Gradually build up your 6 day per week walking times. The 1st week, walk *5 minutes* daily 6 days per week. The 2nd week, walk *10 minutes* 6 days per week. The 3rd week, walk *15 minutes* per day. And finally, by the 4th week, start to walk *20 minutes* every day, 6 days per week. Remember, the speed of walking is not important, unless you are walking too slowly (under 2 mph). The most important factor is that you walk regularly at a relatively brisk pace. If you become tired easily or get short of breath or develop pain anywhere, or if any other unusual symptoms occur, check with your physician immediately. See Medical Precautions at the end of this chapter.

FIT-STEP® STEPS

Our bodies are one of the few machines that break down when not in use. A physically active person is one who is both physically and mentally alert. A walking program can actually slow down the aging process and add years to our lives. Walking has been proven to be a significant factor in the prevention of heart and vascular disease. It strengthens the heart muscle, improves the lung's efficiency, and lowers the blood pressure by keeping the blood vessels flexible. Walking will add years to your life, and life to your years!

In order to walk comfortably and efficiently without tiring, you should balance your body weight over the feet or just slightly ahead of them. Keep your body relaxed, and your knees bent slightly, utilizing a steady, even pace, and a brisk walking stride. To obtain the most benefit out of your walking program you should try to walk with the *Fit-Step® heel-and-toe method,* pointing your feet straight ahead. By utilizing this method, your leg muscles are used more efficiently, and this results in an overall increased blood supply to the peripheral circulation (in particular the legs and feet) and to the general circulation (all of the body's cells, tissues and organs).

The leading leg is brought forward in front of the body, thus enabling the heel of the lead foot to touch the ground just before the ball of the foot and the toes. Your weight is then shifted forward so that when your heel is raised, your toes will push off for the next step. Your arms and shoulders should be relaxed, and they will swing automatically with each stride you take. Before long, you will develop a natural rhythm, pace, and stride as you walk. The Fit-Step® walking method uses the calf muscles to pump the blood up the leg veins back to the heart and lungs, and then out through the arteries to all your body's cells, tissues, and organs. This walking method keeps your body lean and your arteries clean.

When you walk, don't slouch. Walk tall! The way to walk is with your head up, shoulders back, stomach in, and your chest out. Learning to walk tall comes with practice, but after a while, this stance will become a natural part of your Trim-Step® walking style. Your stride is the single most important aspect of your walk.

There is no correct stride length. Stretch as much as you can without straining when you are walking. Thrust your legs forward briskly, swing your arms vigorously and feel your energy surge forth as you walk with the Fit-Step® stride.

Keep your pace steady, never push and don't try to accelerate your speed when walking. If you do get tired after a short period of time, stop and rest and then re-start again at a steady and even pace. Don't rush, just walk at a comfortable Trim-Step® pace. Your rhythm of walking is a condition that will come naturally as you continue your walking program. Keep your body relaxed and your stride steady and even, and your rhythm will develop naturally. Uneven walking surfaces that you encounter will control your rhythm, especially going down or uphill. Don't fight it, just walk naturally and you'll be doing the Fit-Step®.

The Fit-Step® walking method is the ideal weight control and fitness program. Studies in human physiology have proven that walking acts as a weight reduction plan without actually dieting and a fitness program without strenuous exercises. Too often today we allow a sedentary lifestyle to dominate our daily living. We sit at our desks all day and in front of the TV set in the evenings. We drive to our destination, no matter how close or how far, instead of doing what's easy, natural and healthful-walking. Most of us would rather spend 15 minutes in our cars waiting at the drive-in window of a bank, rather than getting out and walking the length of the parking lot. Even at work, we opt for the elevator even if it's only for a few floors. At the supermarket or shopping mall most of us would rather drive around the parking lot several times, so that we can get a parking spot closer to the store. These are all good opportunities to do the Fit-Step®, not the car-step. Use your feet, not your wheels, and you'll look great and feel full of pep when you do the Fit-Step®.

Remember, it's the amount of *TIME* that you walk every day that is more important than the distance or even the speed. If you walk *20 minutes every day,* it doesn't make any difference whether you are walking 2 ½ 3, 3 ½ or 4 miles per hour. You are still burning calories, losing weight, and developing physical fitness. In other words, it doesn't matter how far you walk or how fast you walk, as long as you walk regularly. *You'll be walking 6 days each week to keep your fitness and energy level at its peak.*

TAKE THE NEXT STEP FOR VIGOR, VIM AND PEP

Once you've started walking 6 days per week, you will begin to notice the many changes brought about by your improved aerobic fitness and maximum oxygen capacity (the uptake and distribution of oxygen through your body). You will have lots of pep and energy, a trim figure, improved breathing capacity and muscle tone, improved exercise tolerance, a better night's sleep, a feeling of peace and relaxation, and a lessening of tension. Once you have completed this 4-week conditioning program, you will have taken the first steps towards improved cardiovascular fitness, good health and a long, happy life. Then all you need to do is walk 20 minutes every day except Sunday to reap all of the fitness benefits of the FIT--STEP® PLAN.

The great part about walking as an exercise is that you aren't limited to a particular time or location. Walking doesn't require special clothes or equipment. You can walk before or after work, or if you drive to work, you can park your car a block or two from the office, and walk the rest of the way. If you take the bus or train, get off a stop before your station and walk. An enclosed mall could be the perfect place for your walk in bad weather. Remember to take 20 minutes from your lunch break and walk. Just think of how good that fresh air will feel and smell.

Each city usually has a guidebook containing historical sites, restaurants, shops of interest, cultural centers and interesting walking tours. If you live near a park, the country or the seashore, a walking trip will be a refreshing change. Take the time to walk everywhere. Each new area has its own natural beauty. The wonderful world of walking is literally at your feet. Just take that next step for *vigor, vim and pep.*

INDOOR FIT-STEP® PLAN

Don't wait until the "weather is better" to go out and walk. There's no excuse for not exercising at home on any day when the weather is too cold or windy. Also take precautions against exercising when it's very hot or humid outdoors. Heat exhaustion and occasionally heat stroke are complications frequently found in those crazy jogging nuts that you see running on hot, humid days. Remember, it's not necessary to walk outdoors if the weather is extremely cold, windy, wet, hot or humid. For more information on *weather warnings* see Chapter 9. Here are various indoor exercise alternatives to help you stay on your **FIT-STEP® PROGRAM.**

1. STATIONARY FIT-STEP®:

This is a combination of walking and running in place. Walk in place for 5 minutes lifting your foot approximately 4 inches off the floor and taking approximately 60 steps a minute (count only when right foot hits floor). Alternate this with 5 minutes of running in place lifting your foot approximately 8 inches off the floor and taking approximately 90 steps a minute (again only count when the right foot hits the floor). Use a padded exercise mat or a thick rug. Wear a padded sneaker or walking shoe. Bare feet will cause foot and leg injuries. Repeat this walk-run cycle (10 minutes total) 2 times daily for a total of 20 minutes. If you tire easily, stop and rest. I would rate this exercise - *Boring!*

2. SKIPPING FIT-STEP®:

If you're coordinated enough to use a jump rope, skipping can be a fun indoor exercise. Skip over the rope alternating one foot at a time for 5 minutes and then skip using both feet together for 5 minutes. Use a mat or padded rug with a padded low sneaker or walking shoe. This 10-minute session can be repeated 2 times daily for a total of 20 minutes. If you feel you are not coordinated enough for rope skipping, then *skip it!*

3. DANCE FIT-STEP®:

Turn on the music and dance to your favorite music, whether it's pop, jazz, classical, R&B, or any music with a moderately fast beat. Make up your own moves and dance to the beat of the music. If you can keep it up for 20 minutes, good for you. Otherwise, two 10 minute sessions separated by a rest period will still keep you aerobically fit.

4. STATIONARY BIKE FIT-STEP®:

One of the easiest ways to continue your indoor Fit-Step® program is by using a stationary exercise bicycle. This is the only one-time investment you'll ever need to make as you travel the road towards fitness and good health. No other type of exercise equipment is necessary for your Fit-Step® program.

The most important features to look for in a stationary bicycle are a comfortable seat with good support, adjustable handlebars, a chain guard, a quiet pedal and chain, and a solid front wheel. Most come with speedometers to tell the rate that you are pedaling and odometers to tell the mileage that you pedal. An inexpensive stationary bike works just as well as an expensive one. Stationary bikes with moving handlebars are worthless. They claim to exercise the upper half of your body. In reality, they move your arms and back muscles passively, which can result in pulled muscles and strained ligaments.

The stationary bike is the safest and most efficient type of indoor exercise equipment that can be used in place of your outdoor walking program. You can listen to music, watch TV, talk on the telephone, or even read (a bookstand attachment can easily be clamped onto the handle bars) while riding your stationary bike. If the bike comes with a tension dial, leave it on zero or minimal tension. Remember, it is not necessary to strain yourself to develop aerobic fitness. Exercises like walking and the stationary bike can be fun, without being painful or stressful. You may alternate days of outdoor walking and indoor cycling depending on your individual schedule.

You should pedal at a comfortable rate of between 10-15 miles/hour. To complete your daily exercise requirements, pedal for 20 minutes every day (divide into two 10-minute sessions to avoid fatigue). Always wear a walking shoe or sneaker (never pedal barefoot). A chain guard prevents clothing from getting caught in the bike chain; otherwise roll up your sweats.

5. TREADMILLS:

The treadmill is an effective way to burn calories and build cardiovascular fitness. Manual treadmills are hard on the feet, since you have to push down to make them move and the walking motion is unnatural. Look for motorized treadmills with a deck area (the walking space) with enough length and width to accommodate any stride. The deck area should be at least 18 inches wide by 55 inches long. A cushioned deck is better for your ankles and knees and a thick tread belt is best. You can compare the thickness by the feel when you try out the treadmill or by asking the salesman for the thickness measurement. Look for motorized treadmills with a high continuous duty rating of at least 1.5 horsepower as opposed to a motor with a maximum output. Continuous duty motors give you constant maximum power, whereas maximum output motors surge to accommodate short spurts, but you won't be able to walk smoothly for an extended period of time. You can also choose a treadmill with a power incline; however, too much of an incline is bad for the knees and ankles and can put a strain on your back. Also, make sure that the machine has an automatic stop button, since, if you stumble or feel dizzy, you can push the button and halt the machine instantly.

6. SWIMMING:

20 minutes of swimming provides the same aerobic conditioning and cardiovascular fitness benefits as walking and other indoor Fit-Step® exercises. Swimming, in fact, has the added benefit of being easy on the joints, especially if you have any form of arthritis or back problems. The reason for this is that swimming puts very little stress on the joints because of the decreased gravity factor provided by the buoyancy of the water. If you have access to an indoor or outdoor swimming pool, then 20 minutes of swimming will fit the bill perfectly for the Fit-Step® plan.

7. ELLIPTICAL FITNESS MACHINES:

This type of machine combines the movement of a treadmill and a stair climber. Your feet loop forward to simulate walking, but the footpads rise and fall with your feet. The elliptical motion provides a no-impact type of exercise, which is great if you have arthritis or knee or back problems that make walking difficult. For maximum exercise, an elliptical machine with dual cross-trainer arms, which move back and forth as you stride, rather than the stationary arms, provides maximum exercise and burns more calories and uses more muscle groups. Most of these machines come with an adjustable ramp incline and resistance settings. However, the normal setting is usually more than adequate for cardiovascular fitness. Also, be careful of small space-saving elliptical machines, since they may not comfortably accommodate a tall person's stride, or may not afford full range of motion. Many women, however, complain that the elliptical motion feels unnatural, not at all like walking. They feel as if you have to pull your feet up and then push them down to sustain this motion. Try out different machines to see if you're comfortable with this type of motion. If the motion feels awkward, unnatural or strenuous, forget it.

8. CROSS-COUNTRY SKIER:

This type of machine gives you a workout similar to an elliptical cross-trainer. However, you must be in relatively good shape to be able to work the cross-country skier. The motion is kind of awkward with this type of machine, and in many cases, significantly difficult to use. It is not recommended as an indoor fitness exercise machine for the Fit-Step® plan.

9. ROWING MACHINES:

Rowing machines can provide a vigorous workout and are good for the arms, back, abdomen and legs. However, rowing machines put a significant amount of stress on the lower back muscles and have resulted in many cases of back injuries, including herniated intervertebral discs. This is not a recommended indoor fitness machine for the Fit-Step® program.

10. STAIR STEPPERS:

Since climbing stairs requires more effort than just walking forward, it would seem logical that a stair-stepper would give you an excellent workout. However, the stair-steppers require considerable pressure to move each pedal and puts significant strain on the upper thighs, hips and back. This is not a suitable cardiovascular fitness machine and has been implicated in many types of chronic back and hip injuries. This is not a recommended indoor fitness type of equipment for the Fit-Step® program.

11. RECUMBENT STATIONARY BIKES:

The people who sell recumbent stationary bikes claim that body alignment is more comfortable and natural on a recumbent bike. They also tend to say that the bike seats are more comfortable and ergonomically shaped than seats for upright bikes. Saddle soreness is a big problem for women who ride recumbent bikes, because of the way the body is arched forward. Also, upper back and lower back problems can arise from this unnatural positioning of the body on a recumbent bike. This type of equipment is not recommended for the indoor fitness component of the Fit-Step® program.

12. MALL WALKING:

For those of you who don't like to exercise at home when the weather's bad, an indoor mall can be just the place to take your 20 minute walk. Many malls open early before the stores open to accommodate "mall walkers." If you have access to one of these enclosed malls and don't like to stay at home exercising, then by all means, get out there and do the Fit-Step®. Remember to put vigor, vim and pep into your mall walk step. Keep your eyes straight ahead so that you won't be window shopping instead.

Caution: If any of these Fit-Step® indoor exercises cause excessive fatigue, weakness, shortness of breath, dizziness, headaches, chest pain, pain anywhere in the body or any other unusual symptoms or signs, stop immediately and consult your physician. See Medical Precautions at the end of this chapter.

GET A CHECK-UP BEFORE YOU FIT-STEP®

Even though walking is the safest and most hazard-free exercise known to women, it is still essential that you have a complete physical examination by your family physician before starting your walking program. A thorough examination will usually include a complete physical examination, your personal and family medical history, a resting electrocardiogram, a chest X-ray, complete blood testing, a urinalysis and perhaps a pulmonary function or breathing test, among other tests that your doctor may feel are indicated.

An exercise electrocardiogram may also be recommended for those over 35 years of age and for anyone younger with a family history of heart disease, if your physician thinks that it is indicated. This type of electrocardiogram is taken while you are walking on a treadmill and measures your heart's response to stress while you are exerting yourself. Sometimes this test is combined with an injection of dye (Thallium scan) for a more detailed evaluation of your heart's coronary arteries. Your physician may feel that other heart tests, like a coronary arteriogram or an echocardiogram, may be needed if he suspects that you could have heart disease. It is essential that you follow your own individual doctor's recommendations before beginning any exercise program including walking.

MEDICAL PRECAUTIONS FOR YOUR FIT-STEP® PROGRAM

1. It is essential that you consult your own physician before embarking upon a walking program or any other form of exercise plan whatsoever.

2. If you have a medical disorder that requires that you take medicine or treatment of any kind (e. g. high blood pressure, arthritis, diabetes, etc.), check with your physician before starting upon your walking program.

3. If you develop chest pain, excessive fatigue, dizziness, shortness of breath, pain or discomfort anywhere in the body, stop your walking programs and see your doctor immediately.

4. Avoid any exercise, including walking, immediately after eating. Time is necessary for digestion to occur.

5. Never walk if you are ill or injured. The body needs time to repair or heal itself

6. Avoid walking outdoors in extremely cold or hot weather or when the humidity is above 60%. Use the **FIT-STEP® INDOOR PLAN** as described in this chapter. Always make sure your exercise room has proper ventilation.

7. Do not smoke. Carbon monoxide from smoking decreases the blood's supply of oxygen to the body's cells and tissues. Nicotine narrows the blood vessels, which impairs the circulation. Also don't forget about the risks of heart disease, cancer and lung disease, which are the direct result of smoking.

8. Alcohol should be restricted since it has an adverse effect on the heart's ability to respond to exercise. Many cases of abnormal heart rhythms have been reported from the combination of alcohol and exercise.

9. Anytime you become tired, stop and rest. Don't push yourself. Walking should be fun, not work.

10. Don't exercise before bedtime, since the exercise may act as a stimulant and prevent you from falling asleep.

11. Keep a bottle of water handy, and drink often to keep from getting dehydrated.

12. Your heart rate usually will not exceed 85-110 beats per minute when you are walking. A rapid heart rate is not necessary for physical fitness and good health. If you become short of breath or tired or feel your heart pounding, stop and rest; you're probably walking too fast. *Remember, a walking program at any speed is beneficial for fitness and good health.*

FIT-STEP® WALKING TIPS

1. Be alert. Be aware of your surroundings.
2. Look and listen carefully and observe who is behind and in front of you.
3. Avoid an area that is unpopulated: deserted parks, trails, streets, parking lots, open fields.
4. Vary your route and time of day that you walk. Stick to daylight hours.
5. Walk in familiar or well-populated areas. Plan your route beforehand.
6. If you feel uncomfortable in any area, turn back; follow your intuition.
7. Let someone know where and when you walk. Carry a cell phone or change for a pay phone.
8. If possible, walk with a dog, a friend, or carry a stick, a walking cane, an umbrella, or just a branch for protection.
9. Ignore strangers who ask you questions or call after you.
10. Don't wear radio, tape or cd earphones; they prevent you from hearing traffic or people coming up behind you.
11. Stay away from areas where people may hide: bushes, parked cars or trucks, alleyways, parking lots, etc.
12 If you are threatened or are suspicious of anyone, run into a shopping center, apartment house, crowded street or just knock on someone's door.
13. Wear a whistle on a chain or carry a pocket noise alarm. Don't hesitate to use them even if you just suspect trouble.
14. Wear light-colored clothing, especially if walking at dawn or dusk so that you are easily seen by traffic. When clothing is wet it appears darker than when it's dry, so be careful in rainy weather.
15. Never trust a moving vehicle! They'll never give you the right-of-way. Don't argue with a car. You'll be the loser.
16. Avoid overgrown or wooded areas and dark streets.
17. Stay away from parked vehicles containing strangers.

18. If you become tired, stop and rest in a populated area (example: restaurant or a store).

19. If you're lost, call a friend or the police, never hitchhike.

20. Be bright at night. Wearing reflective material on clothing and shoes while walking after dark or at dusk can mean the difference between a safe walk or a trip to the hospital. Reflective material will increase visibility as much as 200 to 750 feet. According to the American Committee of Accident and Poison Prevention, this reflective material could reduce night-time pedestrian deaths by 30-40%. Be bright at night, don't risk your inner light.

21. And lastly, buy a good pair of walking shoes. Make sure the shoe fits properly. Shoes should be at least ½ to ¾ of an inch longer than your longest toe. The toe section should be wide and high enough so as not to cause compression of your toes. The shank (section between heel and ball of foot) should be wide enough with enough cushioning material to feel comfortable and springy. The upper part of the shoe should be made of materials (soft leather, fabrics, suedes, etc.), which are porous and flexible. The sole and heel should be made of a thick, resilient material which absorbs the shock of walking on a hard surface. And above all, make sure the shoes are comfortable.

22. 10 Tips on Buying Shoes:

 a. Don't choose shoes by their size. Choose them by how they fit on your feet. (Remember, sizes vary among different shoe brands and styles.)

 b. The size of your feet changes as you grow older. It's a good idea to have your feet remeasured regularly.

 c. In most people, one foot is larger than the other. When you go shoe-shopping, have both feet measured. Then select shoes that fit the largest foot.

 d. Try to find shoes that conform as closely as possible to the shape of your foot.

 e. If possible, try on shoes at the end of the day: that's when your feet are their largest and widest.

f. Stand up when you are trying on shoes. Make sure there is enough space between the end of the shoe and your longest toe. "Enough space" usually means that you should have room to put your finger between the end of your longest toe and the end of the shoe.

g. Make sure the ball of your foot fits comfortably into the widest part of the shoe.

h. Don't buy shoes that feel tight, hoping they will "stretch."

i. Select shoes that fit your heel comfortably and that allow a minimum amount of slippage.

j. Walk in the shoes that you want to buy to make sure that they fit and feel right.

FIT-STEP®: IS FULL OF PEP

Many people wonder how exercising actually boosts your energy level and makes you feel energetic several hours after the exercise and have a peppy feeling of well being for the rest of the day. Before I answer that question, let's step back a minute and start with our sedentary couch potato who just begins an exercise program. More often than not, after the first two or three weeks of an exercise program, she complains of easy fatigueability and a general tired feeling after exercising. This is a dangerous time for most exercise participants, because these feelings of fatigue and malaise often lead into a high dropout rate. "I feel worse than I did before I started," or "This is too much for me," or "I can't afford the time it takes to exercise, and I still feel lousy." You should be aware of this critical period at the beginning of any exercise program. If you work on through this feeling, you'll come out feeling more energetic and peppy. It just takes persistence and consistency.

After the first 3-4 weeks, that feeling of fatigue and malaise will be replaced with one of high-power energy and alertness. The reason for the initial delay is the time that it takes the body to develop the physiological changes which makes the production of the energy boosting capacity. These changes range from a more efficient respiratory system to take in and distribute oxygen, to a more efficient cardiovascular system to transport oxygen-rich blood to all of the cells and tissues. This results in a more efficient processing of oxygen and nutrients by the cells of all of the body's tissues and organs. This in turn leads to a more efficient production of energy. Remember, with the *Fit-Step® plan you only need 20 minutes daily 6 days per week for your aerobic fitness level to peak.*

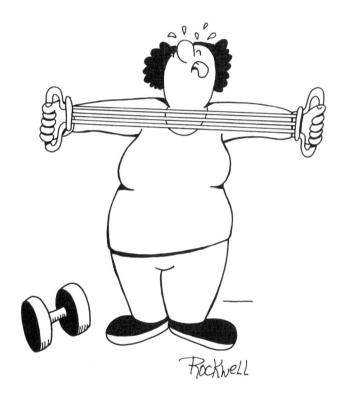

**"THIS LOOKED EASY ON TV.
NOW HOW DO YOU LET GO?"**

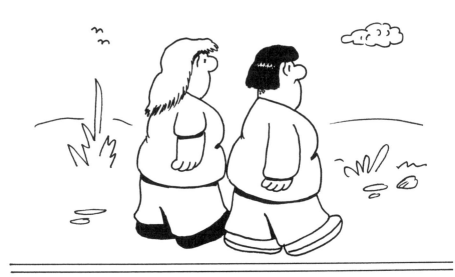

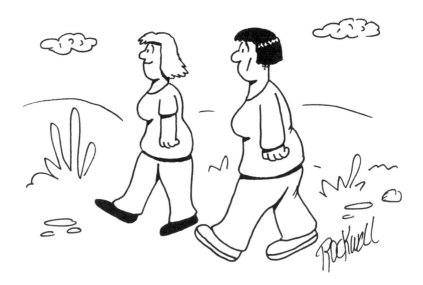

"I DON'T KNOW ABOUT YOU, BUT I FEEL THINNER ALREADY -- AND WE'VE ONLY BEEN WALKING FOR 20 MINUTES."

Chapter 8

WANT TO LOSE WEIGHT FASTER?
****

Women are more likely to perceive themselves as obese, whereas in reality, men are more likely to be overweight. In a recent Harris poll of over 1,200 women and men nationwide, the findings were are as follow:

* Over 50% of women considered themselves overweight compared to 38% of men.
* 65% of the men were actually overweight compared with 62% of the women.
* Almost 40% of those people surveyed stated that they were on a diet.
* 60% of those surveyed were overweight, which was exactly the same percentage as last year's survey.
* More than 50% of those surveyed felt they weren't getting enough exercise.

It doesn't appear that we're getting any thinner despite all of the diet books, health clubs, fitness centers and diet promoters! So what's the answer? Walking, of course! Walkers by and large are the least overweight segment of any population group. This fact has been verified in numerous medical studies.

THE FAT FORMULA

The latest report from the National Institute of Health again confirmed that obesity is a *major health risk*. The evidence is strong that obesity not only shortens life, but actually affects the quality of life also.

Almost 20 percent of Americans are overweight. How can you tell if you're one of them? It's simple-just follow the **fat formula** for your normal weight:

> **Females** - 100 lbs. for the first 5 feet in height, plus 5 lbs. for each additional inch. Example: 5'2" = 110 lbs.
> **Males** - Not an issue!

Body mass index(BMI) is just a complicated measurement which says the same thing. It is another way to assess body fat in relation to your height. Generally a BMI of 25 or more is considered "over-weight", and 30 is considered "obese."

The increased medical risks for being overweight are: *hypertension, heart attacks, strokes, diabetes, arthritis, cancer of all types, and increased surgical risks* if you happen to need an operation. These risks seem to be even worse if most of your weight is carried in the upper body (chest, hips and abdomen) rather than in the buttocks and legs.

If you flunk the fat formula, just **W**alk-**O**ff-**W**eight using the accelerated **Fit-Step® Plan.** Let's put felonious fat where it belongs-- off the street and behind bars.

"I DON'T REALLY EAT THAT MUCH!"

The question I get asked most often from patients about being overweight is, "How come I keep gaining weight? I don't really eat that much." Well, the truth of the matter is that we get heavier as we get older because our physical activity tends to decrease even though our food intake stays the same. The only way to beat the battle of the bulge is to burn those unwanted pounds away. Walking actually **burns calories.** The following table will give you an idea as to the energy expended in walking, which is actually the number of calories burned per minute or per hour **(TABLE I).**

TABLE I

WALKING SPEED	CALORIES BURNED/ MINUTE	CALORIES BURNED/ 30 MINUTES	CALORIES BURNED/ HOUR
Slow Speed (2 mph)	4-5	130-160	260-320
Brisk Speed (3 mph)	5-6	160-190	320-380
Fast Speed (4 mph)	6-7	190-220	380-440
Race Walking (5 mph)	7-8	220-260	440-520

A pound of body fat contains approximately *3,500 calories.* When you eat 3,500 more calories than your body actually needs, it stores up that pound as body fat. If you reduce your intake by 3,500 calories, you will lose a pound. It doesn't make any difference how long it takes your body to store or burn these 3,500 calories. The result is always the same. You either gain or lose one pound of body fat, depending on how long it takes you to accumulate or burn up 3,500 calories.

You can then actually lose weight by just walking. When you walk at a speed of 3 mph for *one hour every day,* you will burn up *350 calories each day.* Therefore, if you walk *one hour a day for 10 days,* then you will burn up to a total *3500 calories.* Since there are 3,500 calories in each pound of fat, when you burn up 3,500 calories by walking, you will lose a pound of body fat. You will continue to lose one pound of body fat every time you complete 10 hours of walking at a speed of 3 mph. It works every time!

WON'T EXERCISE MAKE ME HUNGRY?

Another myth regarding diet and exercise, is that exercise stimulates the appetite. So after exercise you're hungry, you eat more, and you cancel out any calories you burned during exercise. Right? **Wrong!**

Contrary to popular belief, walking actually decreases your appetite. It does this by several mechanisms which are described as follows:

1. Walking regulates the brain's appetite control center (appestat) which controls your hunger pangs. Too little exercise causes your appetite to increase by stimulating the appestat to make you hungry. Walking, on the other hand slows the appestat down, thus decreasing your hunger pangs.

2. Walking redirects the blood supply away from your stomach, towards the exercising muscles. With less blood supplied to the stomach, your appetite is reduced.

3. Walking burns fat rather than carbohydrates and therefore does not drop the blood sugar precipitously. Strenuous exercises and calorie-reduction diets both drop the blood sugar rapidly, and it is this low blood sugar that stimulates your appetite and makes you hungry. Walking on the other hand is a more moderate type of exercise and consequently burns fats slowly rather than carbohydrates quickly. This results in the blood sugar remaining constant. And when the blood sugar remains level, you do not feel hungry.

4. Walking also helps to keep up the resting basal metabolic rate (BMR). This basal metabolic rate refers to the calories your body burns at rest in order to produce energy. When you go on a calorie restriction diet, your BMR slows up. This is because your body assumes that the reduction in calories is the result of starvation and your body wants to burn fewer calories so that you won't starve to death. The body has no way of knowing that you're on a diet. This is also one of the reasons that you don't continue to lose weight on a calorie reduction diet. The body prevents this excess weight loss by lowering its BMR, so that you stop losing weight, even though you are eating the same number of calories that you ate in the beginning of your diet.

If, however, you are combining walking with your diet, then the walking keeps the BMR elevated even though you are dieting. So, in effect, it prevents the BMR from dropping and burning fewer calories, as when you are dieting alone. The result: less hunger and more calories burned when you walk every day, especially if you are also on the Diet-Step® Plan.

WOMEN WHO SAT, DIDN'T BURN FAT

If you just count calories, your chances of losing weight are minimal. *Walking,* however, is the only certain way towards permanent weight reduction. The majority of obese people are much less active than the majority of thin people. It is their sedentary lifestyle that accounts for their excess weight and not their overeating. If they just took a brisk walk for one hour every day they could lose 18 pounds in 6 months, or 36 pounds in one year without any change in their diets.

If you want to lose weight permanently, then the energy burned during your exercise should come from *fats* and not from carbohydrates. During the first 20 - 30 minutes of moderate exercise, only 1/3 of the energy burned comes from carbohydrates while 2/3 comes from body fats. During short bursts of exercise, 2/3 of the energy burned comes from carbohydrates and only 1/3 from body fat. It stands to reason, then, that a continuous exercise like walking, which burns primarily body fats, is a lot better for permanent weight reduction than short spurts of strenuous exercise (examples: jogging, calisthenics, racquetball, etc.).

If you increase the duration of your walking from your regular daily 20 minutes to 30-60 minutes, you will burn more energy from body fats, resulting in faster weight-loss. Once you've lost your weight, you will maintain your weight better by walking *20 minutes every day* than by doing calisthenics or jogging for 15-20 minutes. This occurs because you will be burning a higher proportion of body fats rather than carbohydrates.

Strenuous exercise after a large meal causes the increased blood supply in the stomach and intestinal tract to be diverted to the exercising muscles. This puts a strain on the cardiovascular system, especially in anyone who has a heart or circulatory problem. A calm *walk*, on the other hand, approximately 60-90 minutes after eating, does not stress the cardiovascular system and burns many of the excess calories that you should not have eaten in the first place. It's far better to get up and walk away from that big meal before you overstuff your face. When you physically walk away from the table you are removing yourself from temptation, but even more importantly, you are allowing the fullness control center in your brain to catch up to what's really going on in your stomach. You are actually full, but you don't know it yet. Remember, *eating less and walking more* are the only two ways to lose weight effectively, or, to put it another way - *walk more and eat less!*

W.O.W.! - WHAT A DIET!

Many studies have clearly documented the *weight-loss effects* of exercise. Even more important is that the weight loss caused by walking is almost all due to the *burning of body fat,* not carbohydrates. This weight loss or weight maintenance can be continued indefinitely as long as you walk regularly. You are literally **walking off weight (W.O.W.).**

Not only does walking *before meals* decrease your appetite, but recent studies show that walking approximately 60 - 90 minutes *after eating* increases the metabolic body rate to burn away calories at a faster rate. It appears, then, that walking after eating is another way to lose additional pounds. Never walk, however, immediately after a large meal is ingested.

This burning of calories at a faster rate has been explained as a combination of the energy expended from walking and the calories burned from the actual ingestion of food itself. This is called the *Thermic Effect of Food* or the *Specific Dynamic Action.* We actually burn more calories as we eat because the energy metabolism of the body actually increases 5-10 percent. This doesn't mean that the more you eat the more calories you'll burn. But it is a good reason for *walking 60 minutes after small meals* for additional weight loss. If you want to lose weight at a faster rate, then walk before meals to cut down your appetite and walk approximately 60 - 90 minutes after small meals to burn more calories. Sounds good to me! **W.O.W.! -What a diet!**

FASTER WEIGHT - LOSS WALKING PLANS

THE FIT-STEP® PROGRAM is based on walking at a brisk pace (3 mph) -provided that there is *no change* in your Diet-Step® Plan. This weight-loss program is based upon calories *burned by walking only.* By following **The FIT-STEP® PRO-GRAM,** you will lose additional weight by actually **Walking-Off-Weight!** This faster weight loss occurs because you will be walking more than just the 20 minutes, 6 days/week as on the Diet-Step® Plan.

Three miles per hour is a speed that can be maintained for a long duration without causing stress, strain or fatigue. We are not talking about window-shopping walking which is much too slow (1 to 2 miles/hr) and which is not at all useful in burning calories. Nor are we suggesting fast walking (4-5 miles/hr.), which is too fast to be continued for long periods of time without tiring. And we certainly are not recommending race walking (5 to 6 miles/hr), which is worthless as a permanent weight reduction plan, and has all of the same hazards and dangers that jogging has.

The following walking plans have been designed for *faster weight loss* than the weight loss in the Diet-Step® Plan. You can walk anywhere, any time, any place, as long as you make the time. Remember, you can always take the time to fit a walk into your schedule. And if you don't have the time-make it! Don't wait to lose *weight*, when just walking will make your figure look *great.*

FIT-STEP® WALKING-OFF- WEIGHT PLANS

1. FIT-STEP® PLAN #1 (LOSE ONE ADDITIONAL POUND EVERY 20 DAYS)

On this Fit-Step® plan you will walk for **one hour every other day** or **½ hour every day.** Walking at a brisk pace of 3 mph, you will burn up approximately **350 calories every hour that you walk.** Let's see how much weight you'll lose by this plan.

1. Walk ½ hour daily x 350 calories/hour = 175 calories burned per day.
2. Walk 3 ½ hours per week x 350 calories/hour = 1,225 calories burned per week.
3. Walk 10 hours every 20 days x 350 calories/hour = 3,500 calories burned or one pound lost every 20 days (or 175 cal. burned per day x 20 days = 3,500 calories).

On this walking-off-weight Fit-Step® plan you will lose **one additional pound every 20 days,** or **1½ extra pounds every month.**

2. FIT-STEP® PLAN #2 (LOSE ONE ADDITIONAL POUND EVERY 10 DAYS)

On this Fit-Step® plan you can lose **one additional pound every 10 days** just walking **one hour every day of the week.** The only difference in this plan is that you are now walking an hour every day. You will still be burning up **350 calories** every hour that you walk briskly (3 mph).

Remember, this Fit-Step® plan also works without any change in your Diet-Step® diet plan. Since it takes 10 hours of walking at 3 mph to burn up 3,500 calories or one pound, if you walk for an hour every day, you will lose **one additional pound every 10 days.** By following this plan you can actually lose **3 extra pounds every month.**

3. FIT-STEP® PLAN #3 (LOSE ONE ADDITIONAL POUND EVERY WEEK)

For those of you who want to lose weight even faster, you can walk for **45 minutes twice daily.** By walking a total of 1 ½ **hours every day** of the week you will be able to speed up the walking-off-weight Fit-Step® plan. When you walk 1 ½ hours every day, you will burn up 525 calories each day or 3,675 calories per week. You can see that you will lose a pound a week on this plan with a few extra (175 calories) to spare. You may divide your 1 ½ hours of walking into **three 30 minute** sessions daily if that's more convenient for you. The weight-loss results will be the same. This plan will enable you to lose one **additional pound every week,** or about **4 extra pounds a month.**

Again, all this additional weight loss occurs without your changing one thing in your Diet-Step® plan. By following any one of these 3 accelerated Fit-Step® plans, you will be able to lose more weight than you can lose on the Diet-Step® Plan alone. Remember, it's easy to lose weight and look your best. Just do the Fit-Step®.

4. FIT-STEP® PLAN #4 (FOR CHEATERS ONLY)

Let's say your weight is just where you'd like it to be, but you don't want to gain another ounce. Or say your weight is nowhere near what you would like it to be, but you really can't afford to gain another pound without going into another size dress. Each of you would like to be able to cheat and at least stay the same weight. Well fear no more, the **FIT-STEP® CHEATER'S PLAN** is just for you.

How about a piece of candy, a slice of cake, french fries, a cone of ice cream, a slice of pizza or a glass of wine? With **THE FIT-STEP® CHEATER'S PLAN** you have the perfect method that allows you to cheat without paying the price. Eat your favorite snack food, consult the following table **(TABLE II)** and walk the number of minutes listed in order to burn up the extra calories you've cheated on. The following table shows how many minutes of walking at a brisk pace (3 mph) are necessary to burn up the caloric value of those foods listed.

If your favorite snack food is not listed on the following table, you can easily figure out the time you have to burn off your snack's calories. Look up the number of calories of your favorite snack food and divide by the number 6. This answer will give you the number of minutes it takes to walk off your snack. The number 6 comes from the fact that walking at a brisk pace (3 mph) burns approximately 6 calories per minute. Example: Frankfurter and roll = 300 calories. Divide 6 into 300 and you get 50. It will take you 50 minutes to walk off this snack. "Hot Dog!"

TABLE II

FIT-STEP® CHEATER'S PLAN

BRISK WALKING (3 MPH) BURNS SNACKS

American cheese (1 sl.)	16 minutes
apple (medium)	15 minutes
apple juice (6 oz.)	17 minutes
bagel (1)	23 minutes
banana (medium)	16 minutes
beer (12 oz.)	30 minutes
bologna sandwich	50 minutes
candy bar (1 oz.)	45 minutes
cake (1 slice pound)	63 minutes
chocolate bar/nuts (1 oz.)	28 minutes
cheese crackers (6)	35 minutes
cheese steak (1/2)	55 minutes
chicken, fried (3 pieces)	50 minutes
chocolate cookies (3)	25 minutes
corn chips (small pack)	33 minutes
doughnut (jelly)	40 minutes
frankfurter & roll	50 minutes
french fries (3 oz.)	50 minutes
hamburger (4 oz.) and roll	73 minutes
ice cream cone	30 minutes
ice cream sandwich	35 minutes
ice cream sundae	75 minutes
milk shake, choc. (8 oz.)	42 minutes
muffin, blueberry	25 minutes
orange juice (6 oz.)	16 minutes
peanut butter crackers (6)	50 minutes
peanuts, in shell (2 oz.)	37 minutes
pie, apple (1 slice)	46 minutes
pizza (1 slice)	40 minutes
potato chips (small pack)	33 minutes

pretzels (hard-3 small)	30 minutes
pretzels (soft-1 Superpretzel®)	30 minutes
shrimp cocktail (6 small)	18 minutes
soda-cola (12 oz.)	24 minutes
tuna fish sandwich	41 minutes
wine, Chablis (4 oz.)	14 minutes
Whiskey, rye (1 oz.)	17 minutes

WALKERS WIN BY STAYING THIN!

The question always comes up as to when you should exercise. Is it before or after eating? How long before? How long after? Many professional athletes schedule their day's activities around their meals. Also, many fitness-enthusiasts actually become fanatical and inflexible about the time sequence of exercise and meals. Although walkers don't have to be as particular about timing their walking in relation to meal-time, it's still essential to become familiar, at least in part, with the physiology of digestion.

As food enters your stomach, the heart pumps a significant quantity of blood into the stomach to aid digestion. This does not pose a problem when you are at rest, but if you decide to exercise immediately after eating, then there is a conflict of interests. The stomach now has to compete with the exercising muscles for the blood it needs for digestion. If the exercise gets vigorous then digestion is arrested and you begin to feel bloated and develop abdominal cramps. Exercise should therefore begin after a meal has passed through the stomach and small intestines. This takes approximately 2 - 3 hours after ingesting a large meal and from 60 - 90 minutes after eating a smaller meal.

Foods high in fat and protein are digested slowly and tend to remain in the digestive tract for a longer time than a meal that is higher in complex carbohydrates (whole grain pasta, vegetables, fruits, whole grain cereals and whole grain breads). Foods that are high in refined sugar like cakes, candy and pies can trigger an excess insulin response if they are eaten immediately before exercise. This means that the excess insulin produced as a result of the high sugar content of food, combined with the exertion of exercise, could drop the blood sugar rapidly. This could result in weakness, muscle cramps and even fainting.

On the other hand, fasting for long periods prior to exercise, is in itself counter-productive. In order to replenish the stores of liver and muscle glycogen needed for energy, it is necessary to eat several hours before exercising. With fasting you are depleting these energy stores, and exercise then becomes difficult and tiring without adequate fuel storage reserves for energy.

So what does this all have to do with walking and eating? Very little, if anything. Most of these rules of digestion apply to strenuous and vigorous exercise with relation to mealtime. They do, however, affect us somewhat with regards to our walking program. The most important fact to be learned from this discussion on digestive physiology is that it is essential that you don't walk immediately after eating, especially if you've consumed a relatively large meal (which you shouldn't be eating in the first place). This puts a strain on the cardiovascular system and can even deprive the heart of its own essential blood supply, particularly if you exercise vigorously immediately after eating (which you shouldn't be doing in the second place).

Walking, however, 60 - 90 minutes after a small to moderate meal can actually aid in digestion, by nudging the foodstuffs gently along the digestive tract. This in no way competes for the blood in the digestive tract, since the walking muscles do not pig-out for every available ounce of oxygen like the strenuously exercising muscle-gluttons. In fact, the gentle art of walking allows oxygen to be evenly distributed to all of the body's internal organs, which in this particular case is the digestive tract.

Recent studies indicate a three-fold advantage for dieters who walk before and after meals. As we have previously seen, walking before eating quiets down our appetite-control center in the brain and makes us less hungry. Secondly, walking at any time burns calories directly as we walk. And thirdly, new studies in exercise physiology have shown that walking anywhere from 60 - 90 minutes after eating a small to moderate-sized meal will actually burn 10-15% more calories than walking on an empty stomach. This is explained by a term called *the thermic dynamic action of food*. What this means is that the actual digestion of food-stuffs combined with the gentle action of walking results in a slightly higher metabolic rate, thus burning more calories per hour. You can plainly see how walkers stay thin and full of pep. They just do the *Fit-Step®*.

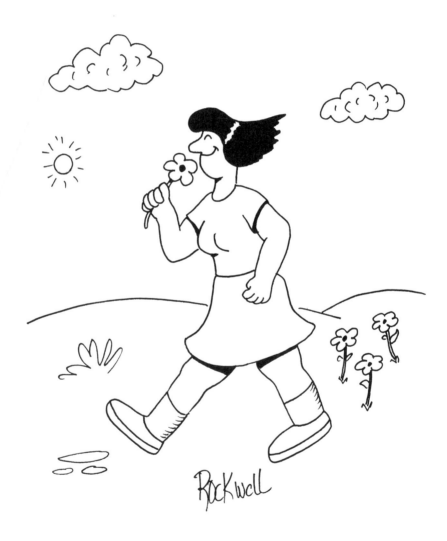

CHAPTER 9

FITNESS, FUN AND FLOWERS
****

SHE WALKS IN BEAUTY
"She walks in beauty, like the night
Of cloudless climes and starry skies
And all that's best of dark and bright
Meet in her aspect and her eyes"
Lord Byron

WALKING WOMEN SEXIER

A new study released at a meeting of the Society for the Scientific Study of Sex, revealed that moderate exercise increases women's sexual drive. Over 8,000 women who exercised regularly were interviewed for this research study. The following are a summary of the findings of this study:

* 98% of women interviewed stated that exercise boosts self-confidence.
* 89% of women reported an improvement in sexual self-confidence.
* 47% stated that their capacity for sexual arousal had been enhanced.
* 39 % reported an increase in making love more often.

The following reasons were postulated for these extraordinary findings. First was that exercise increases the brain chemicals *endorphins,* which are the body's natural chemicals which make you feel good. Walking also acts as a natural anti-depressant and makes you feel better about yourself. Walking also not only makes you feel good but it actually makes you look prettier and healthier by increasing the blood supply to the skin and scalp. Walking regularly also seems to regulate the natural release of female hormones from the ovaries. Whatever the reasons are - *Walking Women Are Sexier!*

THEY CAN'T FOOL ALL OF US ALL OF THE TIME

According to the latest Roper Poll, approximately 50% of the female population stated that walking was their favorite form of exercise. Surprised? Don't be. The fitness industry would like us to think otherwise. That's why hundreds of millions of dollars are spent each year on advertising health and fitness clubs, jogging apparel, aerobic centers, fitness machines and any other gimmicks that these advertisers can use to empty your wallets. Well, take heart America, they can fool some of the women some of the time, but not all of the women all of the time. They won't advertise walking because they can't make a dime from it.

THE PERCENTAGE OF WOMEN WHO REGULARLY ENGAGE IN VARIOUS FORMS OF EXERCISE

Exercise	Percentage
WALKING	46%
CALISTHENICS	16%
SWIMMING	12%
BICYCLING	8%
GOLF	6%
TENNIS + RACQUETBALL	5%
JOGGING	4%
BOWLING	3%

TAKE A HAPPY WALK

Americans are walking again like never before. According to

the President's Council on Physical Fitness report, walking is the single most popular adult exercise in America. With over 52 million adherents, the numbers are steadily increasing as women of all ages are walking for health, fitness and fun. Walking is an exercise whose time has finally come. Why not? It's easy, safe, fun and it makes you feel and look great.

Walking is something that two people, no matter how different their physical conditions, can do together. It is a companionable exercise in which you enjoy each other's company and at the same time get all the benefits of exercising. Walking is a great escape. You can get away from the phone, from the office, or from home for a little while, and take that needed time to relax. You can walk to think out a problem or walk to forget one. Walking acts as a tranquilizer to help us relax and it can work as a stimulant to give us energy. The late famous cardiologist Dr. Paul Dudley White said, *"A vigorous 3 mile walk will do more good for an unhappy but otherwise healthy adult than all the medicine and psychology in the world."* Don't make the common mistake of thinking that walking is too easy to be a good exercise. On the contrary, walking is not only the safest, but it's the best exercise in the world. If you're overweight, then walking is your best choice since you won't be putting excessive stress on the ligaments, muscles, and joints.

How you walk also tells whether you're happy, sad, angry, ambitious or just plain lazy. Walkers with a long stride, a greater arm swing, and a bounce to their step are happy, ambitious and self-assured, whereas walkers with a short stride, foot shuffle or drag and a short arm swing are often depressed, unhappy and angry. Recent studies in women indicate that arm swing is the most indicative factor of their mood. The greater the arm swing, the happier, more vigorous and less depressed a woman is. A short arm swing indicated that a woman was angry, frustrated and unhappy. Stretch out your stride, swing your arms, and put a bounce in your step whenever and wherever you walk. That's your road to good health, a successful career and a long, happy life. Believe it! It works!

WALKING WITCHCRAFT

There is considerable agreement among most exercise physiologists that exercise on a moderate, steady basis has a tranquilizing effect. A rhythmic exercise like walking for 20 minutes seems to be the most effective method for producing this tranquilizing effect. Several theories have been proposed to explain this tranquilizing effect. One current theory is that a slight increase in body temperature affects the brainstem and results in a rhythmic electrical activity in the cortex of the brain. This produces a more relaxed state and is the direct result of exercise. Other studies indicate that there is an increase in brain chemicals, particularly a group of chemicals called the endorphins. These appear to have a tranquilizing or sedative effect and result in relaxation.

In a recent study reported in the *New England Journal Of Medicine,* researchers suggested that regular exercise may increase the secretion of two chemicals called *beta-endorphin and beta-lipotropin.* These substances act as chemical painkillers or tranquilizers and thus can influence the body's metabolism and give a sense of tranquility and well being. This study noted that with exercise, these levels of chemicals increased, and with more strenuous exercise, this increase was even greater. This may, in part, explain the "runners' high" or "joggers' euphoria" that is reported with high-intensity exercise. They stated that this also might explain the frequency with which joggers sustain fractured bones while running without feeling any pain.

Walking, on the other hand, produces only a moderate rise in these brain chemicals. This results in a relaxed state of mind and produces a tranquilizing effect on the entire nervous system. Since walking is not a strenuous exercise, the level of these brain chemicals does not go too high, thus avoiding the analgesic or pain-killing effect produced with high-intensity exercises. This enables the walker to be aware of pain if she turns her ankle or foot while walking. The runner, on the other hand, because of the high analgesic levels of these brain chemicals, may not actually feel the chest pain from a heart attack and she may drop over dead before she becomes aware of the pain. The abnormally high levels of these brain chemicals in this case is another example of too much of a good thing-the devil's deadly draught.

Walking witchcraft, on the other hand, is just the magic you need to fight the devil's sorcery and the voodoo of everyday stress and tension. The calm, serene enchantment of walking (moderate levels of the tranquilizing brain chemicals) fights off the black arts of tension, nervousness, anxiety and stress. *Let the wonderful wizard of walking lead you down the peaceful path of restful relaxation.*

HOW ABOUT A WALK JUST FOR FUN!

Walk whenever you can, instead of driving. If you have to drive, park somewhere a few blocks from your destination and walk the difference. Take the stairs instead of the elevator whenever possible. Take a walk when you are in a new part of town. Always walk when you are away from home to see the beauty of different surroundings. Enjoy your walk by exploring different areas around your home or office, and don't forget to look at the flowers. Take the time to smell the roses, just make sure there are no bees on them. If the weather is bad you can go to an enclosed shopping mall and walk. You can stop and look in all the windows after you've completed your regular 20-minute workout walk in the mall.

You don't have to time your pulse. You don't have to do warm up with stretching exercises before you walk. You don't have to do cool down exercises when you finish. You don't have to tire yourself or get overheated or out of breath. You don't need special clothing or equipment, just a good pair of comfortable walking shoes. You don't have to be an athlete or an acrobat. All you have to do is walk your feet for fun and you automatically, without trying, will stay fit and trim.

HOW NOT TO HAVE FUN!

Thousands of women who have joined fitness clubs in the past have been brainwashed by their so-called fitness instructors into believing the "no pain, no gain" fallacy. They have been intimidated into exercising "until it hurts," or when, at the point of total exhaustion, the instructor says, "Give me five more good ones." And if you want to look fit and trim like the twenty-one year old robotic fitness instructor, you'd better "use it or lose it." Most of these so-called fitness instructors have had very little or no training in exercise physiology, and very few, if any, have been certified or accredited by the American College of Sports Medicine.

In a recent survey of over 1500 women who participated in aerobic classes, over 53% sustained injuries. These injuries included strained muscles, sprained ligaments, torn cartilages, dislocated joints, stress fractures, and even slipped discs. Several cases of stress-induced strokes and heart attacks were included in this list of injuries. These injuries were sustained during strenuous aerobic exercises and calisthenics, and even low-impact aerobic exercises. Most women who engage in these exercises were not sufficiently conditioned to take the excessive strain put on their ligaments, muscles and joints. Once these injuries were sustained, the re-injury rate almost doubled because of inadequate healing time given for recovery in most cases.

Have you ever seen a jogger smile? Of course not. It hurts too much. Runners hit the ground and impact their joints with approximately three to four times their body weight, so it is not unusual that over 60% of runners develop some form of arthritis by the time they're thirty-five to forty-five years of age. The list of potential serious injuries sustained by jogging and other strenuous exercises include musculo-skeletal injuries, including sprains, fractures and dislocations; compressed nerves from slipped discs and various nerve injuries; bladder and kidney injuries; menstrual irregularities and uterine and ovarian damage; heartbeat irregularities, including high blood pressure, heart attacks and strokes; exercise-induced asthma, wheezing, and partial lung collapse; stress ulcers and colon abnormalities; blood-sugar abnormalities and loss of blood minerals (calcium and potassium); heat-exhaustion and heat-stroke; decreased sex-drive and infertility; retinal detachments and eye hemorrhages; anemia and other blood abnormalities; and finally, anxiety, depression and obsessive-compulsive behavior (running mania). *It certainly doesn't sound like they're having fun, does it?*

Walking is kinder to your body and produces better health, fitness and weight-control benefits than jogging or other strenuous exercises without the stress, pain and strain on your body. Medical research has proven again and again that exercise does not have to be painful in order to have beneficial results. The so-called "no-pain-no gain" theory is actually insane. Walking is the only exercise that you can safely continue for the rest of your life for a healthier, happier you. *Walking certainly is the road to fitness, fun and flowers.*

TRAVEL FIT WITH THE FIT-STEP®

Whether you're taking a vacation or a business trip, you can still keep trim and fit with your walking program. Most major airlines, cruise ships and trains offer special diet menus. If you have to splurge on one meal a day, don't worry. You'll walk it off in no time at all. *Cruise ships* and trains are ideal for short walks. Walk around the airport concourse while waiting for flights or during layovers. Most major hotels can give you a map of the area for a walking tour. Get up early before your meeting and take a brisk 20 minute walk. Use the stairs whenever possible and walk around the hotel as much as possible if the weather is bad.

Many hotels have small *gyms* where you can swim or use a stationary bike - take advantage of them if the weather's bad instead of watching TV. Many business trips are associated with a lot of stress and walking can ease away the tension, leaving you more relaxed and more efficient. Speakers always do better after they've had a walk - more brain oxygen and relaxing chemicals (endorphins) and less carbon dioxide result in a sharp, clear, concise speech with no stage jitters. You can keep fit and have lots of pep when you do the **FIT-STEP®.** Don't let a little trip, trip you up. Most people feel exhausted after a vacation or a business trip because they sit around all day and stuff their faces with food and drink. Make it a habit to walk at least 20 minutes every day that you're away. You'll return from your travels fit, full of vigor, vim and pep.

WEATHER WARNINGS

I caution my patients against any kind of physical exertion when the weather is extremely hot and humid or cold and windy. There's no need, however, to stay indoors during mild to moderate changes in weather conditions, since very few of us have perfect weather all year. In fact, if you just wait for that warm, sunny, low humidity day to come along, forget it! You'll never walk. That type of day is never there when you want it. The most important consideration in your walking program is to continue it on a regular basis, day in and day out. *Consistency* is the key word, no matter what the weather is, except in the extreme changes of weather that we will now discuss.

HOT, HUMID WEATHER

Hot and humid weather has its own special set of circumstances. Generally, you have the option in hot or humid weather of being able to avoid these weather extremes by just changing your walking times to early morning or after sunset to avoid the hazards associated with heat and humidity.

When the temperature is above 75% or if the humidity is above 60%, there is the danger of not being able to cool the body off. As we exercise, we expend energy and produce heat. The only effective way to dissipate that heat is by the evaporation of sweat from the body surface. Since *high temperatures* and *high humidity* impair this process, the body temperature will rise. *Radiant heat* from the sun will also increase the body temperature. Even with adequate liquid intake before and after exercise in hot weather, it is still a strain on the cardiovascular system. A walk in the early morning or late evening will avoid most of the problems associated with high temperatures and humidity, and radiant heat exposure.

Heat exhaustion with its rare complication of heat stroke can usually be avoided by the above precautions. There is, however, on rare occasions that extremely hot or humid day when it is even unbearable to walk early in the AM or the late evening. High humidity presents many difficulties with any outdoor exercise program and should be avoided whenever possible. This is the time to quietly and peacefully turn to Chapter 7 on the **Indoor Fit-Step®** program and turn up the air conditioner and relax.

HIGH ALTITUDE

High altitude can also affect your response to exercise, since there is a decrease in the oxygen content of the air. Fatigue sets in more rapidly during exercise since the blood will be transporting less oxygen to the muscles. Caution is advised, especially if you have a pre-existing lung or heart condition. If you fatigue easily or develop difficulty in breathing, then you should stop your walking program. For most people, however, a cautious and gradual approach to exercise here will have no adverse effects.

SINGING IN THE RAIN!

How many times have you looked out of your window at the falling rain and said to yourself, "I wish it would stop raining so that I could get a breath of fresh air." Well, keep looking, the air is still out there. It didn't go away because it started to rain. In fact, the air outside in the rain is actually fresher than it is at any other time. The rain washes away a lot of the air's impurities including pollutants, carbon monoxide and ozone. You'll be surprised how fresh the air smells after being cooped up indoors all day.

So what are you waiting for? Find your umbrella and a pair of rain shoes and go outside and have yourself a truly refreshing walk in air that has been really washed clean. Walking in the rain can be an exciting experience. Look up at the changing patterns of the sky, watch the birds and ground animals, if you can. And above all, smell the air, the grass and the flowers, if they're around. It's a truly unique experience, because it's a time to see, feel and smell nature that I'll bet you've rarely done.

The only precaution that you need to take, is to have an umbrella or waterproof headgear, and waterproof leather shoes or rubber boots or shoes. Also remember to dress warmly if there is a chill in the air. A waterproof raincoat or slicker should be used if you want total body coverage. Be careful not to purchase nylon fabrics that have been coated with a waterproof chemical or plastic, since, although these fabrics keep rain out, they don't let heat and water vapor (perspiration) out. If the garment doesn't breathe in order to let perspiration evaporate, then you could get chilled.

We're not talking about walking in a storm or when it's thundering and lightening. But a walk in a light or gentle rain can be fun and invigorating. If it starts to become a heavy downpour, seek shelter until it lets up a bit. Remember, don't let mild changes in the weather prevent you from your appointed walking rounds.

It's not necessary to go out in all types of inclement weather, like the mail-women have to. But if walking and singing in the rain was good enough for Gene Kelly, then it should be O.K. for the rest of us.

COLD, WINDY WEATHER

The most important consideration in any exercise program is to maintain it on a *regular* basis. However, when winter weather is extremely cold, one should avoid exercising outdoors when conditions are *hazardous*. Walking in the *snow* can be dangerous because you can never tell what type of terrain is underneath the snow cover and injuries are sustained quite easily. Also, icy conditions should be avoided since the danger of slipping and injury are always present. There are many good alternatives to continue your walking program on an indoor basis as you've seen in Chapter 7. If, however, the conditions are such that you feel that you would like to continue your walking program in cold weather there are several precautions that we must mention.

WINTER WALKING PRECAUTIONS

1. If you have any type of *medical condition* (heart, lung, kidney, diabetes, high blood pressure, etc), you should avoid winter walking.

2. If you develop any *symptoms* such as shortness of breath, dizziness fatigue or pain and discomfort anywhere, promptly discontinue winter walking.

3. Follow *medical precautions* outlined at the end of Chapter 7.

4. Dress properly and make sure that you wear extra layers of clothing; heavy *sweat socks or thermal socks, a face or ski mask* may be a good idea, and mittens or ski gloves are helpful.

Mittens keep the fingers together and provide more warmth than regular gloves. Make sure that the *layered clothing* you wear is loose fitting and can be easily adjusted so that you have the ability to open all layers if necessary. If you begin to perspire, you should be able to partially open your clothing so that the perspiration can evaporate. It is interesting to note that you can get up to 100 times as cold in sweat-soaked clothing than in dry clothing.

-*Shoes*-a lined shoe or boot will be particularly helpful in preventing numbness of the toes and feet and will help to preserve the circulation by preventing heat loss.

-A *scarf* over your mouth will warm the air before it is inhaled.

-A *hat* will also preserve body heat (up to 35-40%).

5. *Wind* - Take special precautions with winter wind. Start your walk into the wind, since you should face the worst part of the weather while you are still dry and relatively fresh. If you start your walk first with the wind at your back, you might get overheated and perspired and then when you return and walk into the wind, the perspiration could freeze on your skin with the possibility of developing *frostbite*. Cases of *hypothermia* (the body's inner temperature dropping below normal) have occurred in conditions such as this, where the wind chill factor was such that its effect on a heated perspiring body produced hypothermia, which is a dangerous condition.

6. *Visibility* - It is important to realize that in the winter visibility may be poor and the possibility of auto accidents are increased. Be sure that you wear highly colored bright clothing, especially if you are out after dark, and be sure that you pick a well-traveled route where the automobile traffic is limited.

WINTER WEIGHT-LOSS WALKING

Since winter is the time that most of us usually gain weight, a winter's walk can not only be fun but actually has an added slimming effect for you as a bonus. Walking in cold weather has all the benefits of walking in warm weather with one basic plus - you don't have to walk as long or as far to get the same benefits, in particular the same weight-loss benefit. Since there is more exertion involved when you walk in cold weather, calories are expended more rapidly. Studies show that while a one hour walk at 3 miles per hour burns approximately 350 calories per hour, the same walk on a cold winter day expends close to 400 calories per hour. The basic physiological facts behind this result from the added weight of your clothing necessitated by the cold weather and the subsequent extra effort needed in walking. The result: **MORE CALORIES BURNED PER MINUTE.**

"I'M GIVING UP--EXERCISE IS BORING"

How many times have you heard someone or even perhaps yourself say, *"I'm giving up. Exercise is boring."* Over 65% of women who start an exercise program abandon it after 4-6 weeks. Surprising, isn't it? Not really! Initial enthusiasm is often quickly replaced by boredom. Most of the exercise equipment and athletic clothes quickly find their way into the recesses of the closet.

Walking, fortunately, is one of the only exercises that the majority of women stay with. The percentage of women who give up walking as a regular form of exercise is less than 25% of those who start on a walking program. Perhaps it's because walking doesn't require special equipment or clothing. Or perhaps it's because there are no clubs to join or dues to pay. Or perhaps it's just that most walkers are usually rugged individualists and are more determined than most to keep in good shape.

I think the real reason that walkers stay with their walking program is simply that *walking is fun!* And isn't that what an exercise should be? True, we all want physical fitness, good health, weight control and longevity. But we also want an escape from the stress of every-day living, and that's simply having fun. Walking provides a stress-free, fun-filled activity that we can do anyplace, anywhere, anytime whatsoever. Here are some tips to keep your walking program interesting, enjoyable and most of all, filled with fun.

1. ***Don't expect results too soon.*** Whether it's fitness or weight-control that you're looking for, remember, "Rome wasn't built in a day and neither were you." Give your body time to adapt to your regular walking program.

2. ***Make your walking program convenient and flexible.*** The more adaptable you are to when and where you walk, the more likely you are to do it on a regular basis.

3. ***Vary your walking program.*** Vary your walking times (morn-ing, afternoon or evening) depending on your schedule.

4. ***Change your walking route every week or two.*** If near home or work, walk in a different direction, and observe, feel and smell new sights, sounds and odors on your new route. The road less traveled may be the most fun.

5. ***Keep a record of your walking program.*** For example, how long did you walk today, and approximately how far did you walk? Record the time and location of your walk and your impressions of the area in which you walked. Maybe it's an area you'd like to stay away from or one you'd like to explore again.

6. ***Record your weight only once every week*** to see if you are los-ing the amount of weight you'd like to lose, or if you are just walking to maintain your present weight. Remember walkers who want to maintain their present weight usually can have a bonus snack everyday without gaining an ounce (see Chapter 8).

7. ***Either walk alone or with a friend or relative.*** Walking can be a social activity as well as an exercise. Spending time with someone you like or love can certainly add to the enjoyment of your walking program. Walking is one of the only exercises that lets you talk as you walk. If you are unable to talk because of shortness of breath then you're probably walking too fast.

8. ***Take a walk-break instead of a coffee-break.*** Walking actually clears the mind and puts vitality and energy back into your body's walking machine. Coffee and a donut add caffeine and sugar to your body's sitting machine. Both the caffeine and sugar cause your insulin production to be increased, and following an initial rise in blood sugar, there is a sharp drop in your blood sugar from this excess insulin. So instead of coming back to work invigorated as you do from a walk break, you come back fatigued, light-headed and dizzy from a coffee-donut-break.

9. ***Buy or borrow a dog.*** Studies show that dog-owners who actually walk their dogs have a built- in incentive to stay on a walking program. If you're not a dog person but need a hook to hang your walking program on, there are a number of shops that sell pedometers to keep track of the miles that you walk. Many stores now also carry walking sticks for dress or protection when you walk. These sticks can also help you climb hills if you are hiking and can act as a handy weapon if you have need to use one.

10. ***Don't be afraid to take a break for a few days or even a week.*** Any exercise program, even one as easy and fun-filled as walking can eventually become a little tiring. A few days' break from your schedule will give you a short breather so that you can return to your walking program with renewed interest and enthusiasm. Remember, you won't gain all of your weight back or get out of shape if you take an occasional break from your walking program.

11. ***Never exercise if you are injured or ill.*** Your body needs time to heal and recuperate from whatever ails you. Remember, you can't exercise through an injury or an illness. Many so-called fitness-nuts have tried this with disastrous results. For example, a strained muscle has been aggravated into a fractured bone or a simple cold has turned into pneumonia. Listen to your body. It's smarter than your brain.

12. ***Promise yourself a treat when you stick to your walking program.*** For example - a bouquet of flowers, a night at the theatre, a movie, a candle-light dinner, a new dress or a weekend away. Indulge yourself. You deserve it!

YOUR FUN AND FITNESS CALENDAR

On a cold, crisp, clear January day,
A brisk walk keeps colds and flu away.

Avoid February's bitter, cold chill,
With a walk instead of a doctor's pill.

After deepest winter comes the March thaw,
Which makes walking fun and not a chore.

Don't be afraid of a light April shower,
Take your umbrella and walk for an hour.

Nothing can beat the lovely month of May,
A walk amongst the flowers makes you feel O.K.

You can feel just great in the days of June,
By walking happily and whistling a merry tune.

Even though there's heat and humidity in July,
Don't let an early morning or late evening walk go by.

Don't forget those hot steamy days of August,
An air-conditioned stationary bike is enough for us.

Oh how we love those beautiful days of September,
Those are the walks that we will always remember.

Nothing can be more lovely than October's beautiful trees,
To walk amidst the colorful, spectacular falling leaves.

By the time we feel November's winds a' blowing,
Walkers know it's time to button up and get going.

As December's festive holiday season grows near,
Walk merrily along for good health and good cheer.

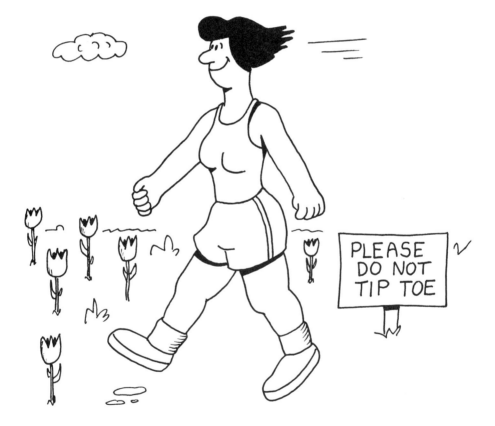

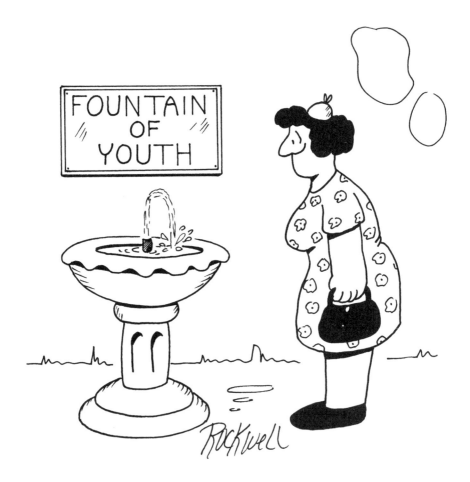

CHAPTER 10

LOOK YOUNGER! LIVE LONGER!
****

THE SECRETS OF THE WALKATHONIANS

In a little known study of a small town in upstate Pennsylvania, walkers appear to live forever. No one has ever reported a death in this community in over 350 years. The elders known as the *Walkathonians* have never allowed any outsiders to view their walking rituals. But legend has it that these *Walkathonians* have been walking regularly for over 350 years and have never developed any disease or disability whatsoever. The only reported deaths have been from falls off the sides of steep mountains and these people have been buried quickly and quietly in order to prevent word of their deaths from reaching the outside world.

It is said that *Walkathonians* feel that their longevity record will be tarnished if any deaths whatsoever are reported. The elder Walkathonian Council has been keeping their written record free of deaths, so that they may qualify for medical notation in either the famous Framingham Heart Study or in the Guinness Book of World Records. Reliable sources stated that they will also be publishing their medical longevity report in a prestigious medical journal later this year. Once the word is officially released, people worldwide will be clamoring for the *Walkathonians'* secrets of eternal life. As one Walkathonian elder told me in a private confidential interview, **"WE JUST WALK!"**

WALK AS IF YOUR LIFE DEPENDED ON IT: IT DOES!

The facts are irrefutable: you live longer and have an improved quality of life if you're a walker. Recent medical studies indicate that walkers live at least 5-10 years longer than non-walkers, and in many cases up to 15-20 years longer.

In a recent study conducted on over 17,000 Harvard school graduates, it was determined that those people who exercised regularly lived significantly longer than those who remained sedentary. Those individuals who exercised consistently had a significantly lower incidence of heart attacks and strokes than those in the sedentary group. And the exercise that most of these graduates reported was -- *walking*. Those that walked the most had the lowest incidence of early death. Walking adds years to your life and life to your years. *Walk as if your life depended on it.* It Does!

DIET-STEP®--LIVE LONGER!

Reducing your daily calorie intake by just 20-25% daily can extend your life by 10-15 years, according to a recent study released by the National Center for Toxicological Research. Based on animal studies, their findings regarding decreased calorie consumption were as follows:

- Extends life and delays the aging process by enhancing your DNA'S ability to repair cell damage that results in disease and aging.
- Slows or prevents cancer by making the metabolism more efficient in eliminating carcinogens from the body.
- Slows the metabolic rate and lowers the body temperature, which in turn slows the aging process.

These findings are based on studies which indicate an apparent delay in the aging process by reducing both the total daily caloric intake and the intake of total fats in the diet. It is essential to provide adequate vitamins, minerals and nutrients in a calorie reduced diet in order to slow the aging process. There must also be a balance between the intake of proteins, carbohydrates and fats. The Diet-Step® plan automatically limits the total calories by limiting the fat content of the diet. It also provides all of the essential vitamins, minerals and nutrients which are essential for good health and longevity.

According to a recent study from Pennsylvania State University, a healthy diet can keep you young. This study found that women 60 to 80 years of age who followed a healthy diet similar to the Diet-Step® diet, had immune systems that function at levels similar to those of women between 20 and 40 years of age. The results show that healthful eating habits may offer a natural means of maintaining the immune system's ability to fight off illness and the onset of degenerative diseases. Walkers, by nature, are usually not big eaters. Perhaps that fact combined with the life-extension benefits of walking is what accounts for the very long life spans of walkers. *Eating less and walking more will give you a long-life for evermore!*

STAY YOUNGER LONGER

Modern medical research is constantly probing the mysteries of the aging process. Molecular biology and genetic engineering are two of the important tools being used by today's scientists in their effort to unravel the complex changes that accompany aging. Since The National Institute on Aging was founded in 1975, research funding has gone from approximately 15 million dollars to over 300 million dollars in 2000. Congress too, like most Americans, wants to live longer and look younger.

The average life expectancy for women is 75.2 years and for men is 70.5 years. Many scientists believe that the life span could easily be extended to well over 100 years if some of the mysteries of the aging process are decoded. After the age of 28-32 the aging process begins to "kick in." These changes first begin at the molecular level in all of the body's cells from the tiniest organs like the parathyroid and pituitary glands to the largest organs like the liver and skin. These changes begin to manifest themselves in a myriad of ways - - graying or loss of hair and wrinkling of the skin; atrophy of the muscles and demineralization of the bones; diminished eyesight and hearing; slight to often imperceptible memory impairment caused by atrophy of brain cells; drooping and sagging skin and muscles; digestive and urinary tract disorders; cardiovascular and respiratory abnormalities; weakening of the immune system and thousands of other subtle changes that accompany the aging process.

Molecular genetics has found that each animal species has a different lifespan, including humans. So what's a body to do? Many people take the fatalistic attitude that their genes will determine when they are to die and that nothing whatsoever can be done to change their genetic code. Nothing could be further from the truth. There are a number of factors that affect the body's immune system, which in turn affects the body's ability to repair damaged or degenerated genes. If, in fact, we can alter the genetic code in a somewhat similar fashion to what scientists do in genetic engineering, then we could conceivably alter life expectancy.

Well, you can do just that! You can stay younger longer. You can live longer younger. You can modify or alter your genetic code and beat the odds against dying an early death or a predetermined genetic-coded death for that matter. The following secrets for breaking the genetic code and beefing up your immune system are:

1. AVOID STRESS TO BREAK GENETIC CODE

Stress produces the release of the hormones *adrenalin* and *glucocorticoids* produced by the adrenal glands. High levels of these chemicals accelerate the aging process by speeding up the death of tiny brain cells and they damage nerve cells throughout the body. These two hormones also produce molecules called *free-radicals* which contain a very reactive form of oxygen. These free-radicals can damage the heart, blood vessels and the lining of the lung. They also have been implicated in the development of certain forms of cancer and arthritis.

Well, how do you avoid stress? It's not as easy as it sounds, is it? Actually it really is. The first thing you have to be aware of is that stress *always wins - - if you let it.* The way not to let stress win is to beat it at its own game. Stress has a lot of henchmen on its side - - adrenalin, glucocorticoids and free-radicals. Well, who do you have on your side willing to back you up every step of the way? Your feet - - that's who! Those two little fellows can beat any combination of adrenalin, glucocorticoids and free radicals twice their size. First of all when confronted with stress say the magic words: *"feet retreat!"* No one has ever beaten stress standing toe-to-toe. If you make the mistaken decision to fight it out with stress, be prepared to go down for the count of ten and then some - - maybe forever! Stress always wins when you confront it head on. The reason is that stress's henchmen, adrenalin, glucocorticoids and free-radicals, have a 1-2-3 punch that's impossible to beat.

Adrenalin speeds up your heart rate and squeezes your blood vessels shut. It causes your pupils to dilate and your skin to become cold and clammy. It shuts down your kidneys and speeds up your intestinal tract. It elevates your blood pressure to dangerous levels making the possibility of a stroke or heart attack likely. Can you beat that 1st punch? Not if your life depended on it!

Glucocorticoids also narrow down your blood vessels and speed up your heart rate. They cause your body to retain liquid which can lead to heart failure. They also cause sodium retention from your kidneys which can further elevate your blood pressure to dangerous levels. They can also damage your kidneys and the adrenal glands themselves, which actually produced the glucocorticoids in the first place. And lastly, they have an adverse effect on your pancreas and can lead to an over-production of insulin which results in sharp rises and falls in your blood glucose levels - - not a good thing at all for your overall health. Think you can duck that number two punch? Not in a million years!

And what about that last punch - - *free radicals*. Free radicals are maverick atoms of oxygen that are produced by the stress reaction. They can cause the deterioration of blood vessels and the alveoli (tissues that line the lungs). They can damage the heart by causing degeneration of the heart tissue. These free radicals, and they really are radical, can cause a decrease in the regular oxygen supply to all of the body's cells and tissues including the heart muscle itself. Without oxygen, organs and tissues die. Without oxygen, heart muscle and brain cells die. These nutty hyped-up oxygen atoms can even cause glaucoma, arthritis and nerve damage. Don't even try to think about beating these crazy little atoms. You'll lose every time.

So what about that secret ingredient I spoke about earlier? *Feet Retreat!* The only way to beat these stress factors (adrenalin, glucocorticoids & free radicals) is to turn on your heels and beat a quick retreat. *Walking away from stress* is your only defense against these dangerous destroyers. Walking away actually dissipates these three killers from your blood stream. As you walk, the levels of adrenalin, glucocorticoids and free-radicals start to decline. The relaxation hormones, beta-endorphins, start to permeate your tissues and cells while the three killer chemicals are pushed out of your blood stream and are eliminated from the body by your liver and kidneys.

Stress is actually a state of mind and if you're willing to succumb to it, you certainly will. If you learn relaxation techniques, like walking, you will learn to deal with stress effectively, rather than letting stress deal effectively with you. A refreshing walk not only dissipates the stress chemicals from your body, but it also dissipates the negative thought processes from your brain. It clears the cobwebs and sweeps the dust out of the corners of your mind. It scrubs clean the walls of your aggressiveness and intolerance. It cleanses the windows of your intellect and it sharpens your mental awareness and understanding, so that you can deal with stress intellectually rather than emotionally. Yes, walking does all that and then some. Try it! It works! Here's a prime example of walking to win, and winning here is more than just winning. It's your life! You can beat stress from within if you *walk to win!*

2. BEEF UP YOUR IMMUNE SYSTEM WITHOUT FAT, REFINED FLOUR OR SUGAR

It's important to select foods that are high in phyto-nutrients, minerals and vitamins and low in saturated fats and refined sugars. Eat more whole grains, fruits, vegetables, fowl and fish and less meat and dairy products. Sound familiar? Of course, it's the Diet-Step Plan. Foods high in saturated fats are particularly harmful to the immune system. These foods raise blood cholesterol levels which clog the arteries and subsequently slow down the flow of oxygen-rich blood and vital nutrients to the body's cells and tissues. This process actually shortens your life expectancy by allowing your vital organs and tissues to die a slow, painful death. No organ can live without adequate supplies of oxygen and nutrients. High-fat foods also take considerably longer than other foods to convert to energy. Eating a high fat meal diverts blood and oxygen from the brain to the digestive tract, leaving you feeling fatigued and lightheaded. Blood cholesterol levels can also be lowered by eating more fruits, vegetables, fowl and fish and reducing consumption of meats, dairy products and pastries, especially those made with palm or coconut oil. The fiber in beans, legumes and oat bran lowers cholesterol as well as the pectin in fruits such as apples, oranges and grapefruit.

Refined sugar and flour play havoc with the immune system by triggering sudden rises in insulin production, which results in dramatic sharp drops in blood glucose levels. This condition known as hypoglycemia can result in fatigue, headaches, fainting spells, weakness and even convulsions. Not only is the body deprived of essential glucose for energy and metabolism, but the brain is also deprived of essential glucose which is necessary for brain function. If the brain cells are deprived of glucose for any length of time, then some of these brain cells may atrophy or die. Like oxygen, these brain cells need a constant infusion of glucose to enable the neurological network to function properly. Once deprived of glucose the brain exhibits memory loss, incoordination, speech impairment, generalized muscle weakness, and even convulsions if glucose deprivation persists for a long period of time.

3. ADEQUATE VITAMINS, MINERALS AND PHYTO-NUTRIENTS

Remember when we spoke about the arch villains called the free-radicals? Well, a diet high in yellow and dark green vegetables provides phyto-nutrients like beta-carotene, which is a precursor to vitamin A. This chemical beta-carotene breaks up free-radicals and protects the body against their harmful effects such as cancer and degenerative diseases. Likewise, vitamin E (a fat-soluble vitamin), found in many cereal grains, fish and non-fat dairy products also protects against the villainous free-radicals. An adequate supply of vitamins C and B-complex are also essential to keep the immune system in good working order. These water-soluble vitamins are essential for good health and longevity. Fruits and vegetables provide an excellent source of these vitamins; however, they must be continuously supplied to the body, because being water-soluble, they are excreted rapidly by the body. A daily vitamin and mineral supplement with B complex, vitamin E and vitamin C is recommended to keep the body's cells and tissues constantly supplied with these essential nutrients. These phyto-nutrients, vitamins and minerals are responsible for keeping the immune system in good working order and they help the body to repair its own DNA (material that makes up your genes). Fruits, vegetables and whole-grain products present in the Diet-Step® diet provide the body with all of the essential nutrients, vitamins and minerals to keep the immune system in tip-top condition.

4. BEAT FATIGUE AND INCREASE ENERGY

a. Sleep

Most people require between 6 - 8 hours of sleep per night. Some individuals need less, others need more. If you wake refreshed in the AM and don't tire easily during the day, then you're probably getting enough sleep. The sleep/wake cycle is affected by many things. One in particular is the release of a hormone called cortisol. This hormone decreases before bed-time and starts to rise in the early AM hours before you awake. Travel and shift-work can effect your sleeping cycle by interfering with the cortisol blood levels. Your body usually will adjust to time changes after several days, by changing the rise and fall of cortisol production. If, for some reason, you are unable to get adequate sleep at night, then a ½ hour nap in the afternoon will leave you feeling refreshed.

b. Smoking

Smoking causes fatigue by impairing the uptake and delivery of oxygen to the cells of all of your body's organs. Smoking increases the level of carbon monoxide in your blood stream, which damages the heart and lungs leading to cardiovascular disease, pulmonary disorders and cancer. Smoking destroys Vitamin C in the body which impairs the immune system and decreases your energy level. Also, smoking causes premature wrinkling of the skin and a sallow complexion.

c. Caffeine

Excess caffeine consumption causes marked fatigue after the initial stimulating effect of the caffeine wears off. Caffeine also has an adverse effect on the cardiovascular and nervous systems. It can cause a rapid heartbeat, palpitations, elevation of blood pressure and an irritation of all of the body's nerve endings. This can result in headaches, nervousness, sweats, tremors, mental confusion, anxiety and even paranoid behavior. Following these adverse effects comes marked lethargy, sapping the body of its vital energy.

d. Salt

Excess salt intake can cause a permanent elevation of blood pressure by interfering with the kidney's ability to eliminate salt from the body. This excess accumulation of sodium causes the body to retain more liquid and subsequently increases the volume of blood. This in turn makes the heart work harder causing a rise in blood pressure. In susceptible people this may result in permanent hypertension and premature death from strokes or heart attacks.

e. Alcohol

Excess alcohol can cause liver disease, brain damage, nerve disorders, strokes, heart disease, hypertension, damage to the reproductive organs, spleen enlargement, hemorrhages of the esophagus, liver and pancreatic cancer and early death. This is certainly not the road to looking younger and living longer.

f. Keep mentally active: Think young!

As you age, you can expect fatigue and a dulling of the mental senses unless you keep mentally active. Keeping mentally active requires that you continuously stimulate the brain cells by reading, doing puzzles, playing games such as checkers, chess or cards, keeping up with or learning a new hobby or skill or constantly interacting with other people. By keeping mentally alert you will stay younger longer and enjoy your years with less fatigue and more energy and pep. Remember, it's important to think young! Staying young is as much a state of mind as it is a state of body physiology.

5. STOP SEDENTARY SITTING

Inactivity is associated with obesity, diabetes, hypertension, heart disease, pulmonary and gastrointestinal disorders, arthritis, back problems, muscular and mental tension and premature death. Walking, on the other hand, increases the delivery of oxygen to the brain and body tissues which improves the circulation. This results in increased energy and mental alertness. Walking also decreases stress and tension, thus producing muscular and mental relaxation. This in turn lowers the blood pressure and prevents cardiovascular disease. Walking also lowers the LDL (bad cholesterol) and raises the HDL (good cholesterol), protecting you from heart disease.

Walking burns calories and prevents or controls obesity and diabetes. Walking builds muscle and bone tissue and prevents osteoporosis, arthritis, and degenerative muscular and neurologic disorders. Walking prevents the development of chronic lung disorders by keeping the lungs and respiratory muscles in good working order and by preventing the lung capacity from shrinking.

Walking boosts the immune system by producing chemicals known as *interferons* that do everything from warding off colds to preventing cancer. In fact, when you come right down to it, walking helps to prevent almost every known disease and disability known to modern science. And above all, walking helps to prevent premature death and even mature death. Walking will allow you to live years beyond your pre-determined genetic-coded death. Population studies show that walkers *live at least 10 - 15 years longer* than their sedentary counterparts.

Women walkers, by and large, live at least 10-15 years longer than sedentary women. Walkers in every country in the world have been proven to be the longest-living segment of any population of any civilization. From the Masii natives in Africa to the Russian tribes in Siberia; from the mountain climbers of Peru to the Bushman of New Guinea; from the train-women in London England to the mail-women of the United States. All of these women have one thing in common - - *they're all walkers!* And for all intents and purposes they live longer than any other similar-age group of sedentary people in their respective cities or countries.

Dr. Alexander Leaf, Professor Emeritus, Clinical Medicine, Harvard Medical School, studied various populations throughout the world and concluded that the active segment of each population had a longer life-span than the inactive segment. He stated - *"It is apparent that an exercise like walking throughout life is an important factor promoting well-being and longevity. One is never too old to commence a regular program of exercise and once started, will never grow too old to continue it."* Walkers live longer and are illness-free longer than their sedentary counterparts anywhere in the world. This was the conclusion reached at the last national convention on *Clinical Research on Aging.*

ANTIOXIDANT SUPPLEMENTS: NOT ALWAYS IN FOODS OR PILLS

Among the many health claims regarding antioxidant supplements, there has been little discussion in the way that the body itself combats damage caused by *free radicals*. Living cells have evolved a variety of internal systems that offer protection against oxidative stress (the term commonly used to describe free radical attack). Oxidative stress is an imbalance between the factors that cause oxidation and the factors that inhibit oxidation in favor of oxidation. The basic cause of oxidative stress is the formation of free radicals. Free radicals are the culprits which make the body's metabolic system and organs' systems break down. It is important to understand how the body protects itself against free radical attacks.

There are many selected antioxidant nutrients that are found in primary food sources, for example, fresh fruits and vegetables, grains and oils, yeast, and many other food groups. The nutrients range from vitamin C, vitamin E, carotenoids, coenzyme Q1O, glutathione present in liver, and many other phyto-nutrients, vitamins and minerals. Here is a surprising addition to the list of agents that affect the body's oxidation process: regular exercise can influence the equilibrium between antioxidation and oxidation, or the oxidative balance. In other words, *regular exercise acts as an antioxidant* just like any dietary or food supplement, helping the body to rid itself of free radicals.

The following is an interesting comparison of the different types of physical exercise when studied at the molecular level. Physical activity influences oxidative balance but it does so paradoxically. During acute phases of physical activity, for example strenuous exercise, more oxygen is needed to create energy; therefore, more volatile oxygen molecules are formed. During this type of strenuous exercise, highly reactive hydroxyl radicals can overwhelm the body's antioxidant systems, and cause injury to the surrounding cells and tissues. Hence isolated strenuous exercise produces significant oxidative stress. However, when physical activity is recurrent or moderate (for example, a walking program), exercise induced oxidative stress decreases over time as the internal antioxidant systems begin to adapt. Thus, regular exercise improves oxidative balance. This is a very complicated way of stating, on a molecular level, what we have been stating all along, in that *strenuous exercise is hazardous to your health, whereas regular exercise, like walking, is beneficial to your health.*

Regular aerobic exercise, such as walking, may improve the oxidative balance in several ways. One way is that it improves the antioxidant protection by regulating enzyme systems that are responsible for cleaning up escaped free radicals. Secondly, it probably decreases resting levels of free radical formation. To put it another way, sedentary people tend to have poor oxidative balance because they undergo oxidative stress even at relatively low levels of physical functioning, whereas fit people tend to have good oxidative balance, because they limit oxidative stress during exercise and during daily functioning. So, the next time you remember to take your dietary antioxidant, whether in food or supplement form, remember to continue your walking exercise program to obtain additional antioxidant protection against those nasty free radicals. *The result is that you'll look younger and live longer.*

WINNING STEPS TO LIVING LONGER

How long you live depends partly on your genetic code. Heredity does play an important role in your longevity factor. However, you can beat your genetic code if you eliminate most of the risk factors of heart disease, hypertension, vascular disease and cancer. The following simplified list is an outline of what you can do to eliminate many of the risk factors that are present in our everyday lives. **Here are 13 steps to living longer:**

1. Decrease salt in your diet to help prevent or lessen the risk of hypertension and stroke.
2. Maintain normal weight to prevent the risk of hypertension, heart disease, obesity, and diabetes.
3. Decrease cholesterol in the diet to lessen the chance of heart attacks, strokes, and blood clots.
4. Decrease saturated fat in the diet to lower blood cholesterol in order to prevent strokes and heart attacks, and to lessen the risk of breast, prostate, and colon cancer.
5. Increase the fiber in your diet to lower cholesterol and to prevent the development of obesity, hemorrhoids, varicose veins, diverticulitis, colon cancer and many degenerative diseases.
6. Increase consumption of green and yellow vegetables which have high concentrations of phyto-nutrients and vitamins A & C to prevent various types of cancer.
7. Avoid the use of smoked meats and smoked fishes which have high concentrations of nitrites that lead to stomach and esophageal cancer.
8. Avoid the use of excess caffeine which can lead to breast cysts, breast cancer, pancreatic cancer, prostate cancer, nervous disorders, heart disease, and high blood pressure.
9. Avoid the use of tobacco which can cause oral cancer, lung cancer, emphysema, hypertension and heart disease.
10. Avoid excess alcohol consumption which may contribute to

liver cirrhosis, liver cancer, hepatitis, pancreatic tumors, heart disease and neurological disorders.

11. Avoid prolonged exposure to the sun to prevent the development of skin cancer.
12. Avoid stress whenever possible to prevent the body's stress hormones from raising your blood pressure and constricting your arteries.
13. *Walk every day to keep aging at bay.*

In addition to these thirteen steps, make sure that you have regular check-ups with your family physician. Be sure to carefully follow any recommendations that she/he has as to your diet, exercise, medications, etc. If you're ever in doubt as to your doctor's advice, don't hesitate to get a second opinion. The worst thing that you can do is to ignore your doctor's recommendations. Also never be afraid to ask her/him questions about things that bother you. And never, ever ignore any unusual signs or symptoms that you develop. Check with your doctor immediately. Don't hide your head in the sand like an ostrich hoping that these symptoms or signs will go away by themselves.

There is no segment of the population that could benefit more from a walking program than the elderly. A younger woman can increase her physical fitness 15-25% by exercising; an older woman may be able to improve her physical fitness 35-50%. As our population gets older, more people are realizing the benefits of regular moderate exercise. In a recent national poll, it was found that over 50% of women 65 and older walk regularly every day.

Walking can reverse or slow down the ravages of the aging process as we have previously seen. Walking helps to control weight, lower blood cholesterol and decrease body fat. Walking helps to build bone structure, strengthen ligaments and tendons, and increase muscle mass and strengthen muscle tissue. Walking helps to condition the lungs and respiratory muscles and improves your general overall breathing capacity. Walking also helps the cardiovascular and circulatory systems by improving the efficiency of the heart's pumping action. Walking helps to keep the blood vessels elastic, preventing the development of hypertension. Walking keeps the blood circulating and prevents the formation of blood clots by preventing the blood platelets from sticking together.

And finally, walking helps to improve the maximum oxygen uptake which increases the oxygen uptake from the atmosphere, its distribution through the blood stream and its final delivery to the cells of the body's organs and tissues. This *improved oxygenation at the cellular level is the basis for the life process itself.* If you can provide a constant infusion of oxygen on a regular basis at the cellular level, then you can slow down the aging process. By providing this oxygen to the cells, your body can operate its cellular machinery more efficiently. The body's cells can utilize the nutrients they receive from the blood stream more efficiently when they are saturated with oxygen, and they can give up their waste-products easier for elimination from the body. *Walking the Fit-Step® way keeps you looking young and can help you live a longer, healthier, happier life.*

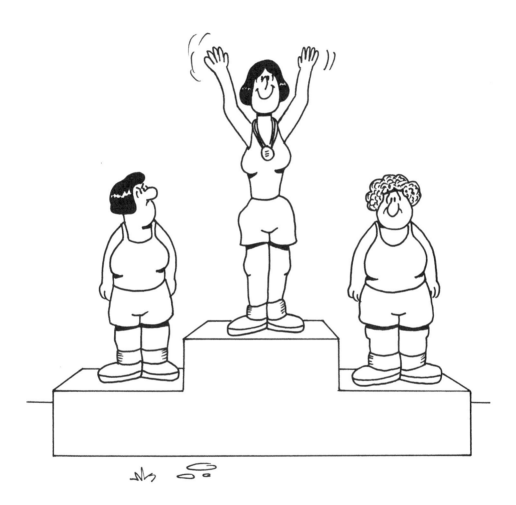

WALKING WOMEN WIN!

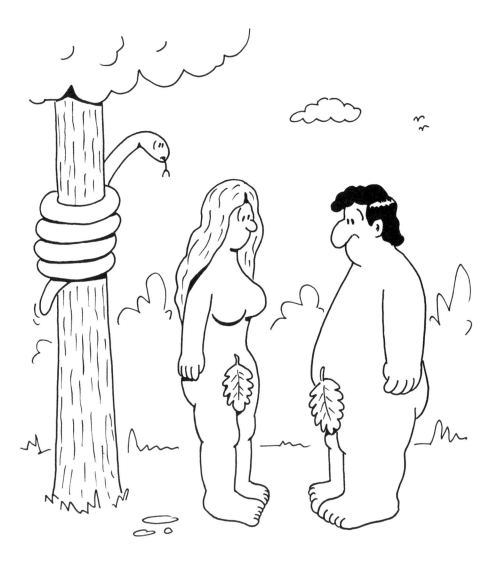

CHAPTER 11

YES, WOMEN ARE DIFFERENT FROM MEN!

****

"Yes, Women ARE Different From Men" was the first page headline in The Medical Tribune (Dec. 1999, Vol. 40, No. 21). Finally new research has discovered that there are significant differences in the physiology of women and men. These differences extend far beyond the obvious reproductive biological differences. These differences affect almost every organ system in the body, including the heart, brain, digestive tract, nervous system and even the skin.

With reference to the heart, women's hearts beat faster at rest than do men's hearts. Also, the electrical behavior of the conducting tissue in the heart is different in women and men, which may explain the normal difference in the EKG's of women and men. It has also previously been found that a woman's coronary arteries are smaller than those of a man. These factors have to be taken into consideration in the diagnosis, treatment and prevention of heart disease in women. Physicians are just beginning to recognize these differences in treating women with coronary artery disease.

Men's brains are larger than women's brains; however, women's brains contain more neurons (nerve connections), which may explain why women are better at multi-tasking (juggling more things simultaneously in their lives:work, child care, home responsibilities, social activities and caring for their big-brained mates). Face it, women are different from men, and smarter, too.

A long held fallacy in medicine has been that whatever medical research that was done on male patients could be interpreted as being the same for women. Nothing could be farther from the truth. For example, women metabolize certain medications differently from men, which must be taken into careful consideration when treating female patients. Many diseases and medications affect women differently, and therefore, these differences must be taken into consideration when formulating different types of treatments for various diseases. Yes, women are really different from men, and it's about time that the medical establishment is becoming aware of that important difference. And isn't it about time that engineers and architects also begin to realize these differences, and start putting more stalls in the restrooms in restaurants, movies, theatres and other public places for women?

Many of these differences in physiology may explain the difference in the fitness response to exercise in women. The maximum oxygen uptake is defined as the highest rate at which oxygen can be taken up from the atmosphere and utilized by the body during exercise. It is frequently used to indicate the cardio-respiratory fitness of an individual. Even though men have a larger overall muscle mass than women, women have more long-term endurance capacity. This may in part be explained by a woman's ability to sustain her maximum oxygen uptake longer by steady, consistent exercise. Men, on the other hand, frequently engage in short bursts of energy expenditure like jogging, racquetball, strenuous weight lifting, etc. This type of strenuous activity does not increase the maximum uptake capacity (uptake and distribution of oxygen throughout the body) for a long enough time to develop maximum aerobic fitness. Women, on the other hand, develop aerobic fitness more slowly than men; however, their fitness and endurance levels are more consistent and long lasting. In other words, women who engage in moderate exercise activity like walking, swimming, stationary bike, treadmill, etc. are more likely to stay aerobically fit than men. In this chapter, we'll see how these differences relate to heart disease, hypertension, stroke, stress, and vascular disease, among others.

"NO PAIN - NO GAIN" - NOT TRUE!

Finally, recent medical research on heart disease is stating what I've been telling my patients and readers for the past 20 years: that moderate exercise prevents heart disease. I've always contended that exercise doesn't have to be stressful, painful or exhausting in order for it to be beneficial. In my previous books, I've refuted the exercise enthusiasts who followed the mantra "no pain - no gain" with reference to fitness development. This theory is pure baloney! Strenuous, painful exercise regimes are no more effective than moderate walking at 3 miles/hr in order to develop cardiovascular fitness and good health. In fact, strenuous exercises are more likely to do more harm than good.

I've also stated over and over again to my patients and in my books that the so-called "target heart-rate zone" is just a myth! No one has ever proved scientifically that a rapid heart rate is essential for cardiovascular fitness. In fact, it could be extremely dangerous to keep the heart beating rapidly for a long period of time, especially in individuals who have undiagnosed pre-existing heart disease. The most important proven fact is that strenuous exercise is not only hazardous, but it is counter-productive to cardiovascular fitness and good health. Strenuous, short bursts of exercise contribute nothing towards the prevention of heart disease and strokes, and in fact, strenuous exercise may actually cause a heart attack or a stroke! These potentially serious consequences may be the result of strenuous exercises raising the blood pressure to dangerous levels or by causing the heart to beat irregularly (cardiac arrhythmias).

In a recent study of over 17,000 women and men, it was concluded that *moderate exercise* is an independent factor in the prevention of deaths by cardiovascular diseases. The following findings were presented by the American Heart Association:

* Despite blood pressure, cholesterol or age, moderate exercise has an independent effect in preventing heart disease and strokes.

* Men in the lower 20% of physical fitness had a 50% higher incidence for heart disease than men falling between the 30-50% range of fitness development.
* Women in the bottom 20% zone of fitness, however, had a 70% higher incidence of heart disease than those women in the 30-50% range of fitness development.
* The major conclusion was that "just a little bit of exercise" is all that is needed to lower your risk of cardiovascular diseases, especially in women. And I think it is a bit ironic that the report ended with my long standing quotation: *"You don't need to run a marathon in order to reduce your risk of heart disease."*

Researchers at the Disease Control Center in Atlanta revealed a startling finding after reviewing 43 previous studies on heart disease. The one statistically significant, predisposing factor in the development of heart disease which appeared in every single study, was a *lack of exercise.* Their research revealed that people who exercised the least had almost twice the risk of developing heart disease as those who exercised regularly. This particular study brought together the findings of the 43 previous studies, which had all measured physical activity in many different ways. Walking was as effective as any other type of exercise in preventing heart disease without the added risk of injury and disability, which occurred in more strenuous exercises. This analysis suggests that the lack of exercise on its own may be as strong a risk factor for developing heart disease as high blood pressure, smoking and high cholesterol. The Disease Control Center also stated that about 59% of adults in the USA get little or no exercise at all. Don't sit around and get obese. *Otherwise you're at risk for heart disease!*

WOMEN AT RISK

Coronary heart disease is responsible for over one-half million deaths each year in the United States. It causes more deaths each year than all forms of cancer combined. There are over 5 ½ million women and men who have been diagnosed as having coronary artery disease. It is estimated that there are at least 2 ½ million other Americans with undiagnosed coronary heart disease, many of them under the age of 50. It has also recently been shown that pre-menopausal women are more at risk for heart disease than was previously thought. The misconception was that only post-menopausal women were at risk because of their lack of estrogen.

In a major hospital study of over 350,000 hospital patients, researchers found that women between the ages of 30 to 40 were more than twice as likely to die after suffering a heart attack as men of the same age. In another study, women of all ages were more likely to develop complications after having had a heart attack than men. Women also may have less typical symptoms when sustaining a heart attack, making diagnosis more difficult. Physicians need to pay closer attention to atypical cardiac symptoms in women. Doctors also need to be more aggressive when it comes to treating women who have heart attacks. It took this long for physicians to finally realize that *women are different from men.*

Coronary artery disease is caused by the build-up of fat deposits in the arteries (atherosclerosis). This disease begins slowly, early in life, and usually doesn't produce symptoms until middle age. This build-up of fat in the arteries, also known as plaque, is of particular importance in women whose coronary arteries have a smaller diameter than the coronary arteries in men. Unfortunately, this condition often goes undetected until a woman has her first heart attack, which may in fact be fatal. Although we have made great strides in the treatment of heart attacks, the emphasis must rest on preventing this slowly progressive disease (atherosclerosis) from occurring. It is estimated that more than 60 billion dollars is spent each year in the treatment of coronary heart disease and less than a million dollars yearly is spent on the prevention of this disease. Physicians need to realize that women's symptoms need to be taken more seriously and that more extensive work-ups should be done on women with suspected heart disease.

In order to prevent or slow the progress of atherosclerosis

we must be aware of the *10 risk factors* which contribute to the development of this disease. One risk factor that we can't control is heredity; however, those people who have a strong family history of heart disease should pay particular attention to the risk factors that we can modify. The 9 risk factors which we can control ourselves or with medical treatment include: **cigarette smoking, excess alcohol consumption, excess caffeine, obesity, high blood pressure, high blood cholesterol, diabetes, stress and inactivity.** One risk factor increases your risk of a heart attack by 25%. If you have two of these risk factors, it increases your likelihood of getting a heart attack by 35%. Three will increase your chances by 45% and four will increase your risk by 55-60%.

How would you like to be able to eliminate or reduce almost all of these risk factors in one fell swoop? There is no need to worry about these risk factors if you start walking like your life depended on it. Believe me, it does! *Walking* can actually help you remove or reduce these risk factors to a minimum with a little additional help from your willpower. How is this possible? The body that exercises doesn't want or need to *smoke* or drink *alcohol* or *caffeine*. The woman who walks stays at her *ideal weight*. Walking lowers your **blood pressure** and your *blood cholesterol.* If you're a *diabetic* or have diabetic tendencies, walking helps to improve and regulate sugar metabolism. Walking is a sure-fire method to ward off the evils of *stress* and *tension*. And, finally, walking every day completely eliminates the coronary risk factor of inactivity. When you Fit-Step®, you are beating the odds against all 9 risk factors of heart disease.

KEEP YOUR ARTERIES CLEAN WITH A WALKING MACHINE

A 52-year-old female executive came to see me recently because of pain in her calf muscles when she walked. She was not able to walk more than a block before severe pain in one or both calves caused her to stop walking. After a few minutes of rest, the pain subsided and she could resume walking again. However, after walking another block or two at the most, the pain resumed and she was forced to sit down again. This patient had a history of moderate hypertension and she had smoked 1-½ packs of cigarettes every day since she was 20 years old. The diagnosis was relatively simple. The patient exhibited all of the classical symptoms of *intermittent claudication.* Vascular studies of the lower extremities confirmed this clinical diagnosis.

Intermittent claudication is defined as pain or cramps in the legs, usually the calf muscles, brought about by exercise (usually walking) and relieved fairly promptly by rest. This condition results from an occlusion (obstruction) in the large and medium-sized arteries leading to the legs. This obstruction comes from the build-up of deposits of cholesterol (atherosclerosis) inside of these blood vessels. As this obstruction becomes more severe, the blood supply to the exercising leg muscles cannot be met. Since these muscles cannot get enough oxygen, they cry out with pain (intermittent claudication) due to the lack of oxygen-rich blood. When the exercise (walking) is stopped, the muscles require less oxygen, so that as soon as a limited blood supply reaches these muscles with some oxygen, the pain stops.

The very first step in the treatment of this condition is to stop smoking. *Carbon monoxide* from smoking promotes atherosclerosis in both the coronary arteries and in the peripheral arteries (those leading away from the heart, for example, legs). Carbon monoxide molecules actually jump into the seats on the red blood cells that were reserved for the oxygen molecules. Without its passenger, oxygen, the red blood cells carry this deadly enemy (carbon monoxide) throughout the body. These carbon monoxide molecules get off at various stops along the arteries to do their dirty work. The arteries that are waiting for oxygen get a big surprise. They get molecules of carbon monoxide instead. This carbon monoxide irritates the artery's inner lining (intima) and subsequently makes it an ideal seeding bed for deposits of cholesterol. Nicotine from the cigarettes also contributes to piling up more cholesterol in the arteries. It accomplishes this by raising the blood pressure, narrowing down the artery's opening (lumen) and by promoting clot formation in the arteries. When you stop smoking you can prevent atherosclerosis from progressing and in some cases you can actually reverse the process.

The simplest and often most effective treatment for this condition is -- yes you guessed it -- walking! "Now wait a minute," you're thinking. "He just told me that walking is what caused the pain in intermittent claudication." That's absolutely correct. However, most medical authorities feel that a gradual walking program is the best form of conservative therapy for this condition. Patients who have stopped smoking and engaged in a modified walking program have been able to double or triple the distance that they can walk without pain. This occurs because walking dilates or opens arteries, making more room available for blood to reach the muscles. Walking also makes more oxygen available to be carried to the arteries. This extra oxygen prevents cholesterol from being deposited in the arteries and it supplies more nourishment to these oxygen-starved muscles. And walking helps to keep the arteries elastic, so that they can stretch and recoil, thus helping to propel the blood along its way.

Finally, walking improves the flow of blood to these muscles by opening up a reserve group of blood vessels that normally just sit in the wings like understudies in a play. These reserve blood vessels are referred to as the *collateral circulation*. Walking actually calls forth these small little-used reserve blood vessels, much the same as the trumpeter calls forth the cavalry. These small vessels located in the legs open up with regular walking and send the blood around (bypass) the blocked arteries. A regular walking program can help to keep these collateral vessels open permanently.

Walking also can actually help to eat away at the cholesterol deposits that have accumulated in the blocked arteries. It accomplishes this by supplying oxygen-rich blood to these blocked arteries and by raising the "good" (HDL cholesterol), which carries these cholesterol deposits out of the body. Walking also lowers the "bad" (LDL cholesterol) in the blood, making less cholesterol available to block up the arteries. If, however, this disease has progressed too far, then medical treatment may be required. Several new drugs that help to open the arteries and decrease the blood's thickness (viscosity) are now available. If these medications are not effective, then surgery may be necessary.

There is a similar type of condition in which cholesterol deposits accumulate in the arteries of the neck (carotid arteries). This form of atherosclerosis obstructs the flow of blood through these arteries and results in a decrease in the supply of oxygen-rich blood to the cells of the brain. This decreased blood supply can lead to a condition referred to as transient ischemic attacks (TIA's). These are actually temporary small strokes with no permanent damage. These attacks can cause visual loss, speech impairment, weakness or partial paralysis of an arm or leg, memory loss, headaches and other neurological symptoms. These symptoms usually last a few seconds to several minutes and then the patient is normal again. Some cases have been known to last several hours. If this process of atherosclerosis progresses to a point where the carotid arteries are almost completely blocked, then vascular surgery may be necessary to prevent a full-blown stroke from occurring.

The best treatment for both of these conditions is to prevent them from occurring. Always check with your physician if you develop any symptoms that you think might be caused by these disorders. The risk factors for developing these diseases are the same as the risk factors for developing heart disease. Cigarette smoking, high serum cholesterol, inactivity, stress, excess caffeine and alcohol, obesity, diabetes and hypertension, all can be modified or improved by walking. Remember, *walking helps keep your arteries clean with your walking machine.*

WALKING AROUND KEEPS BLOOD SUGAR DOWN

Walking may help both Type I diabetics (insulin dependent) to reduce their insulin requirements, and Type II diabetics (non-insulin dependent) to reduce their oral medication dosage. This occurs because walking not only burns calories including sugar, but walking increases the body's cells sensitivity to insulin. Type I diabetics therefore may need less injections of insulin and Type II diabetics become more sensitive to the production of their own body's insulin and may require less oral medication.

A diabetic normally has increased risk factors for heart attacks and strokes. Walking appears to reduce these risk factors by controlling blood sugar, decreasing serum cholesterol, making the blood less likely to clot, reducing total body weight and by opening the tiny capillaries that feed blood to the extremities, organs, tissues, cells, and to the heart muscle itself. An exercise program for the diabetic requires careful medical supervision. All patients should get complete physical exams before starting any exercise program. For most diabetics, that means complete blood-testing, urinalysis, chest X-ray, EKG, and in some cases, a stress EKG. The patient's physician will actually determine what type of tests are necessary. Medication dosages (insulin or pills) should never be changed without a physician's approval.

In general, strenuous exercise should be avoided because it may accelerate sugar absorption which could result in sudden hypoglycemia (low blood sugar) which could result in fainting spells or other serious complications. This is particularly true if a diabetic attempts to exercise too soon after a meal. At least 60-90 minutes should elapse before a diabetic begins exercising. The beauty of a walking program is that it is a moderate aerobic type of exercise without any of the hazards of strenuous exercise. This is especially important in the female diabetic, since she is particularly vulnerable to the side effects of strenuous exercise. Walking avoids the sudden drops in blood sugar that so often accompany strenuous exercise. Walking eliminates the high-impact stress on the nerve-endings and blood vessels of the feet, which are particularly vulnerable in the diabetic to injury from high-impact sports. Walking gently burns calories thus lowering blood sugar moderately. This enables the diabetic to possibly lower her dosage of insulin or oral medication, after the body gradually adjusts to the wonderful world of walking. *Walking keeps your feet on the ground and your blood sugar down.*

WOMEN WHO ONLY SAT FOUND IT FATAL TO GET FAT

In the majority of cases, obesity results from too little exercise and too much food. Life insurance studies have shown that excess weight causes cardiovascular disease with increased mortality. These same studies also reveal that life expectancy improves following weight reduction. Obese people have a significantly higher incidence of hypertension than non-obese persons. The excess body weight demands a higher cardiac output (pumping out blood) to meet the increased metabolism of an overweight woman's body. This in turn causes the left ventricle chamber of the heart to gradually enlarge because of this extra workload. The combined effect of obesity, hypertension and heart enlargement may eventually lead to heart failure and death. Weight reduction can lower both the systolic and diastolic blood pressures if it is accomplished before the complications of heart enlargement and heart failure occur. These medical conditions must always be treated and monitored by your own physician.

Obesity also causes an alteration of the body chemistry and metabolism. The blood sugar goes up dramatically with obesity, often leading to the development of diabetes. The uric acid in the blood becomes elevated, often leading to kidney stones and attacks of gout. Obese women have higher levels of triglycerides (sugar fats) and the "bad" LDL cholesterol. They also have lower blood levels of the "good" HDL cholesterol. These altered blood fats can eventually lead to severe coronary artery disease. These abnormal blood chemistries can be reversed to normal levels, if weight reduction occurs before permanent complications result. And if all these risks of being overweight weren't bad enough, here's another piece of fat not to chew on. *Obesity just by itself has been listed as an independent risk factor for coronary heart disease.* Newer data from the 26-year follow-up statistics in the *Framingham Heart Study* demonstrated that obesity just by itself was enough to cause a significant increase in the risk of coronary heart disease and premature death in both women and men.

There are two extremely effective methods to win the war against obesity. One is to follow the Diet-Step®: 20 Grams Fat/20 Grams Fiber diet plan. The other is to follow the Fit-Step®: 20 minute exercise program. They effectively reduce your weight, including your cholesterol, and they reduce your risk of cardio-vascular and cerebro-vascular disease. Two important steps to *add years to your life and life to your years.*

WALK AWAY FROM TYPE A

Emotional stress can precipitate heart attacks in women with no known history of heart disease. Type A behavior (high-strung, aggressive personalities) has also been associated with an increased incidence of coronary heart disease, completely independent of other coronary risk factors. And patients who already had known coronary heart disease with Type A behavior were shown to have more severe artery involvement than did patients with heart disease who had Type B behavior (non-aggressive, more relaxed type personalities). In today's corporate America, fast paced executives with type A personalities can be found just as often in women as in men. By climbing the corporate ladder, women have also climbed into a high-risk category for strokes and heart attacks. Women also have the added stress of juggling work, home, child care, social responsibilities and many other life events.

New research has demonstrated that emotional stress can cause coronary disease as well as aggravate it in patients who already have heart disease. And all of these studies also show that by reducing stress, both coronary heart disease and hypertension can often be prevented in normal patients and controlled in patients who already have heart or blood pressure problems. Type A behavior can be modified with stress management techniques. These techniques include personal counseling, meditation, avoiding stressful situations, and our true-blue, loyal friend, walking. Walking has been proven over and over again to significantly reduce stress and tension, alleviate anger and hostility, decrease fatigue and malaise, and control anxiety and depression. *Walk away from stress today and your heart will be O.K.*

TURN OFF THAT DAMN COMPUTER!

Why do we always feel as if we need to take a trip or change our environment when we're fatigued or stressed? Why do we say? "Let's go to the beach" or "Let's take a trip to the mountains?" Why is it that after a hard week at the office, you feel like "just getting away from it all." In other words, why don't we just stay put or stand still? What makes us want to get up and go? What inner force is responsible for this feeling that we must seek solace in the great outdoors, someplace away from our present confining environment?

Science has tried to come up with answers to these questions and has made some startling discoveries. Our bodies give off electromagnetic waves like animals, fish and birds. This electromagnetism is what makes birds migrate every year. It is what enables fish to swim upstream to spawn. It is what makes bears know when to hibernate and then when to awaken again. Electromagnetic waves, in fact, govern many of the physiological, biochemical and psychological functions of all living things.

Women, like all other animals, are also governed by

electromagnetic forces that cannot be seen, heard, felt or touched. They can't be studied with a microscope or a stethoscope. They can't be seen in the retina of the eye with an ophthalmoscope. Nor can they be studied in any way known to medical science. Yes, we can evaluate brain waves on an electroencephalogram, and we can study the brain's structure and architecture with a brain scan or an MRI. These electromagnetic forces, at the present time, are not measurable by any known machine or instrument.

All we know is that when a certain amount of tension builds up in our bodies we have to release it. "We've got to get out of the house." "We've got to get away from the office." "We just have to get away for the weekend." "We must get out and take a walk." Our bodies are screaming at us to release the tension. These so-called electromagnetic impulses are telling our nervous systems to shut-down the terminals. Stress is beginning to short-out our bodies like a faulty fuse. The synapses (connecting points) in our brains are becoming inundated with messages of stress and tension. The neu-rons (nerves in the brain and spinal cord) become overloaded like telephone wires with too many calls coming in at the same time. Whether we call this burn-out, or over-load syndrome or just high-anxiety, the message is clear. Our bodies are telling us something. The message is loud and clear, like an SOS from a sinking ship. *"Unplug yourself from the electric current." "Turn your terminals off" "Shut down your nuclear reactor before you have a melt-down!"* ***"And for god's sake, turn off that damn computer!"***

Don't wait for a stroke or heart attack to occur before you start to follow the voice on the e-mail airway of your electromag-netic waves. Don't wait until you've had a major ulcer attack, to lis-ten to the message sent on the electrical impulses of your brain. You must get away now! You must heed your body's inner voice. You must go to where you will feel healthier, happier and refreshed. This is nature's way of protecting you from self-destruction. You can prevent your body from exploding into the atmosphere by get-ting away from stress and tension as often as possible.

Walking increases relaxation hormones in the brain (endor-phins) and decreases stress hormones (epinephrine and nor-epi-nephrine). You will notice how much better you feel almost imme-diately after your walk. Refreshed, relaxed and relieved, you'll be better able to return to the stresses of everyday living with a new perspective on life. You will actually have built-up a type of immu-nity to the tensions that formerly tore you apart. This immunity, like the immunity to certain diseases, needs to be reinforced. *Walking the Fit-Step® way will keep stress at bay.*

FEET ON THE GROUND, KEEPS BLOOD PRESSURE DOWN

According to the American Heart Association, more than one out of every four people in the United States has high blood pressure and the incidence is higher in women than it is in men. Among people age 65 years and older, approximately two out of three people suffer from hypertension. There are approximately 57.7 million Americans who have high blood pressure according to the Heart Association Council for High Blood Pressure Research. Many of these people are at considerable risk for developing strokes, heart attacks, heart failure and kidney disease, unless they receive medical treatment. Women are particularly vulnerable to the complications of hypertension. Unfortunately, many women with high blood pressure have no symptoms and may have hyper-tension for many years before it is diagnosed. Remember; always get your blood pressure checked regularly. And if you already take high blood pressure medication, take it regularly according to your physician's recommendations.

Many cases of mild hypertension may be able to be con-trolled without the use of medication. These methods include weight reduction, salt restriction, cessation of smoking, alcohol restriction, decreasing saturated fats and cholesterol in the diet, stress reduction and exercise. It should be pointed out that the majority of studies on the benefits of exercise for lowering blood pressure, have used walking as the best moderate intensity exercise for this purpose. Jogging and other strenuous exercises can actually raise blood pressure during the actual exercise.

Two major studies reported in a recent issue of the *Journal of the American Medical Association* proved without a doubt that regular exercise, particularly walking, can decrease the risk of developing heart disease and high blood pressure by more than 50%. The first report studied over 6,000 women and men who had no previous history of high blood pressure. Over a period of 4 years, people who did not exercise regularly ran a 52% higher risk of developing hypertension. The second study followed 17,000 women and men over a period of 16 years. Those who exercised regularly experienced only one-half the death rate from heart disease and hypertension. This study showed lower blood pressures and lower death rates, particularly in women who walked regularly.

In no fewer than five other separate studies in hypertensive women and men, a walking program produced lowered blood pressure in over 80% of these patients. The period of exercise training varied in these different studies from three months to three years. It was interesting to note also, that if any women dropped out of the program, their blood pressure gradually went up to its former hypertensive level after six-eight weeks. This confirmed the theory that in order for exercise to be beneficial, particularly for high blood pressure, it must be carried on for a lifetime. And what better exercise than walking can be done for the rest of your life?

There are several physiological mechanisms responsible for the blood pressure lowering effect of exercise. They include improved cardiac output of blood, decreased peripheral vascular resistance to the flow of blood, slower pulse rate, dilation of small arteries, thinning of the blood and a reduced release of catecholamines and angiotensin (the hormones that cause high blood pressure). The fact remains, however, that no matter what the physiological reasons are, walking lowers your blood pressure.

All you have to remember is that if you keep walking with your feet on the ground, you'll keep your blood pressure down!

DON'T STROKE OUT!

Strokes are the third leading cause of deaths in the United States each year. The most frequent contributing factor is high blood pressure. Approximately 65% of all strokes occur in people who never knew they had high blood pressure or in people who had hypertension but did not take their medication regularly. Women are particularly vulnerable and may develop strokes from unregulated or untreated hypertension.

High blood pressure speeds up the process of atherosclerosis (hardening of the arteries). Untreated hypertension damages the lining walls of the arteries and allows fatty deposits to collect in the arteries. This in turn sets the stage for blood clots to form in the blood vessels of the brain, which can cause a stroke. High blood pressure also can weaken the walls of the blood vessels so that a balloon (aneurysm) forms. The combination of high blood pressure and extreme physical exertion (example: strenuous exercise, power-lifting, etc.) may cause this aneurysm to rupture, which results in a hemorrhage into the brain producing another form of stroke.

Fortunately, stroke-related deaths have declined by almost 45% in the United States in the past 10 years. This is due primarily to the widespread, successful treatment of high blood pressure. People are beginning to realize that they have to continue taking their high blood pressure medicine indefinitely, in order to prevent strokes from occurring. Stopping smoking also is important in preventing strokes from occurring. The carbon monoxide from smoking damages the blood vessel walls, and speeds up the process of atherosclerosis. The early treatment of diabetes and obesity also helps to slow down this process of hardening of the arteries, which leads to hypertension and stroke. Also reducing salt and stress helps to lower blood pressure and in turn reduces your risk of stroke.

According to most medical authorities, a moderate program of regular exercise is extremely important in controlling high blood pressure and in preventing strokes. You heard it -- **moderate exercise!** Walking is the exercise most often prescribed by physicians to control hypertension. Walking lowers the blood pressure and can help to prevent strokes. The following steps show you in detail how the Fit-Step® Plan actually lowers your blood pressure, prevents heart disease and strokes, and prolongs your life.

LADIES' LUNCHEON LIMITS

According to the Framingham, MA Heart Study, high levels of triglycerides (often called sugar-fats) may increase the risk of heart attacks and strokes. It seems that the body converts triglycerides into low-density lipo-proteins (LDL's), the so-called "bad" type of cholesterol. The LDL cholesterol is the type that clogs up your arteries and can make you prone to developing either a heart attack or a stroke.

Women seem to be more at risk than men for developing heart attacks and strokes from high triglyceride levels. Men, on the other hand, seem to be more at risk for strokes and heart attacks when their cholesterol levels, rather than their triglyceride levels, are high. Triglyceride levels usually go up when excess refined sugars are consumed, like cakes, candies, pies, ice cream, etc. Women who usually eat more sweets than men seem to develop higher triglyceride levels, since the body's metabolism converts excess sugar into triglyceride. If you have to limit your luncheon desserts don't cry, because *triglycerides may make you die.*

Now for the good news. Walking lowers both triglycerides and LDL cholesterol. So when you sit down for coffee and cake, go

light on the cake and remember to get up and walk those triglycerides off, before they walk their way into your heart for a long
unhealthy stay.

LEGS THAT ARE TRIM, KEEP YOUR VEINS IN

Once your blood has circulated throughout the arteries,
supplying oxygen and nutrients to all of your body's cells, it must
return to the heart and lungs for a fresh supply of oxygen. The
blood must pass from the arteries into the veins before it can be
returned to the heart and lungs. Except for the blood returning to
the heart from the upper third of the body, the return of all the rest
of the blood to the heart from the lower two-thirds of the body must
go upwards against the force of gravity. This flow of blood through
the veins back to the heart is assisted by the contraction of your *leg
muscles* when you walk. The leg muscles actually squeeze the
blood up the veins against gravity. This upward flow of blood is
also aided by the small *one-way valves* located inside the walls of
the veins. These valves actually prevent the blood from falling back
down the veins.

Many women unfortunately have genetically weak veins.
These women are prone to develop varicose veins. Prolonged sitting builds up the venous pressure in the leg veins, which is caused
by the pooling of blood. The excessive pressure that builds up in the
veins actually balloons out these weak veins. This, in turn, stretches out the walls of the veins, and the small valves located inside the
walls of the veins lose their resiliency. After a period of time these
weakened veins permanently dilate (enlarge), and their valves no
longer are able to prevent the flow of blood from dropping back
down the veins. This results in what is commonly called *varicose
or incompetent* veins, which are unable to return all of the blood
back to the heart. Sometimes fluid leaks out of these veins into the
tissues of the legs causing edema (swelling of the feet and legs).

After you have been sitting for a long time, especially when traveling, your circulation slows down. This is why your feet often swell after a long trip. The upward flow of blood from the leg veins can also be impaired by constrictive clothing or by crossing your legs, which causes further swelling in your feet and ankles. Always make it a point to walk around on a plane or train. Make frequent stops when riding in a car to stretch and exercise your legs. Walking will start your leg's muscle-pump working, so that it squeezes the blood up your leg veins and back into your heart for re-circulation. *Walking will keep your legs trim and hopefully keep your veins in.*

One in four adults has vein problems and women are four to ten times more likely to develop them. Varicose veins are twisted and enlarged veins that are typically close to the surface of the skin but can affect deeper veins as well. Crossing the legs is a bad habit and is one of the first things you should learn to undo, if you suffer from varicose veins. Crossing the legs slows the upward flow of blood and increases the pressure inside the veins. It doesn't matter if you cross your legs at the knee or the ankles, both are bad; however, knee crossing is probably worse.

Almost half of all women over the age of 40 suffer from varicose veins or spider veins, which are less serious breaks in smaller, surface veins. The cause is unknown, but genetics is a key factor. Many women develop varicose veins during pregnancy because of increased pressure in the veins, which reduces the valves' ability to close. Diet, obesity, age and a sedentary lifestyle also can contribute to developing varicose veins.

Walking is the first and most important thing you can do to keep your veins strong and healthy. Women who sit 6 - 8 hours per day with their legs crossed will have a greater chance of developing varicose veins if there is a genetic factor. Always take walking breaks during the day. Rotate your ankles and flex your toes while sitting. Eat a high fiber diet to avoid constipation, which increases the pressure inside the veins and maintain your ideal weight on the

<u>Diet-Step® Plan.</u> If you have varicose veins wear mild compression stockings, if your job requires that you stand for long periods of time in one place. Surgery is sometimes necessary if these veins become worse. Always check with your own physician regarding the best treatment for you, if you develop varicose veins.

WITH CHILD - TAKE IT MILD!

The so-called fitness experts have been telling pregnant women for the past 10 years that exercise is beneficial for them. Magazines, videotapes and books have been giving the some messages loud and clear - "It's okay to exercise vigorously when you're pregnant, you'll have a healthier baby." Well, guess what? This advice is all wrong. Recent animal studies show that strenuous exercise during pregnancy may be potentially harmful to the fetus. This apparently happens because of two reasons. First, strenuous exercise may redirect the blood flow away from the uterus and placenta toward the mother's exercising muscles and skin. Any decrease in the blood's supply of oxygen to the developing fetus can be hazardous, causing birth defects, miscarriages, premature births and even fetal deaths.

Secondly, strenuous exercise causes an elevation of the body temperature in a pregnant woman. This rise in temperature is transmitted through the bloodstream to the fetus. This elevated temperature may cause damage to the fetus's developing nervous system resulting in neurologic birth defects. Recent studies in humans have verified these experimental animal studies.

Pregnancy itself makes greater demands on the cardiovascular and muscular system, so it stands to reason that physical exertion should be limited. Strenuous calisthenics, especially leg exercises, strain the ligaments supporting the uterus. And pregnancy causes a woman's center of gravity to shift, making a fall or injury more likely while exercising. Most physicians, I'm sure, would agree that walking is the safest, most beneficial form of exercise for at least the first half of your pregnancy. Always check with your own physician before embarking upon any exercise program, even walking.

WALKING WOMEN WIN WAR!

Women who began exercising and playing sports as young girls appear to develop body changes that reduce their risk of breast and uterine cancers. In a recent study at Harvard School of Public Health these findings were presented based on the fact that exercise in young girls delays the onset of menstruation by several years. The early onset of menstruation is a potential risk factor for developing breast cancer. Active young women have fewer and more irregular menstrual periods which usually reduces the production of female hormones. This may be responsible for the decreased risk of both uterine and breast cancer in exercising young women.

Women who continue their exercise program into later life have less body fat and more lean muscle mass. These women also tend to eat a low-fat diet throughout their adult years. It is a known fact that excess saturated fat makes excess estrogen, which increases the risk of breast cancer. In this study of over 5,000 women, it was also found that the lean women produced a less potent form of estrogen, which was not as likely to cause breast and uterine cancer as was the more potent form of estrogen produced by heavier women. These findings showed that sedentary women had a 2½ times greater risk for developing cancer of the uterus and twice the risk of developing breast cancer. *Walking women win war against cancer.*

Women who remain active during their adult years were also found to have a lower risk of developing heart disease. Walking regularly contributes to the production of a less potent form of estrogen. When this type of estrogen is combined with the hormone progesterone which is naturally produced by the ovaries, active women have lower levels of total cholesterol and higher levels of HDL (the "good" cholesterol).

WALK, DON'T SIT--LET'S MOVE IT!

A recent study at the State University of New York in Buffalo has now linked even colon cancer to lack of physical activity. This condition had been previously thought to be caused only by a *low-fiber, high fat diet.* Now, however, it appears that women with sedentary jobs are 60 percent more likely to get cancer of the colon compared to women with more physically active jobs. In this study, women who had spent more that 20 years in completely sedentary jobs had twice the incidence of colon cancer as compared to those women with active jobs. And women who worked at low-activity jobs had 1½ times the risk of colon cancer as active workers.

Physical activity, especially a regular *walking program,* appears to stimulate the movement of waste products through the colon, thus decreasing the time that the potential waste carcinogens are in contact with the wall of the colon. This is a similar theory to that which explains why a *high- fiber, low-fat diet* also helps to prevent colon cancer. Remember, Diet-Step®: 20 Grams / 20 Minutes is for women only. And like the energizer bunny, it keeps on working, working, and working.

A WALK EVERY DAY KEEPS ARTHRITIS AWAY

Recent research suggests that walking may be the best exercise for most forms of arthritis. Most people with arthritis can benefit from a regular exercise program according to the majority of rheumatologists. And the exercise that most of these doctors recommended for their patients with arthritis was walking. Walking strengthens the muscles and ligaments that are attached to the arthritic joints. This helps to relieve the pain that occurs when the bones rub against each other. Walking also may prevent some of the joint inflammation and deformity that is associated with arthritis. The gentle joint motions of walking may relieve joint pain and swelling. Just make sure that you take it easy and rest frequently. Don't walk through pain.

The recurrent pain and joint swelling associated with arthritis may cause depression in many patients with arthritis. Depression, in turn, leads to lethargy and inactivity. The inactivity, instead of relieving the pain, in most arthritics tends to lead to more joint involvement and greater immobility. Walking, on the other hand, with its biochemical and psychological mood-elevating effects, acts as a natural antidepressant in the arthritic patient. Walking does wonders to improve the arthritic's feeling of well-being and it improves the vicious cycle of pain, depression and subsequent immobility.

Any patient who has some form of arthritis must be monitored closely by their personal physician. Each patient is an individual and will respond differently to various forms of exercise. Just as complete inactivity may lead to a worsening of arthritis, too much activity, especially strenuous exercises, may also have an adverse effect on arthritis. Listen to the advice of your own physician. Most doctors, however, will recommend a graduated walking program for the majority of their patients. *Don't let pain keep you in. Get out there and Walk to Win!*

WALK AGAINST DEPRESSION

In a recent issue of <u>The Physicians and Sports Medicine</u> it was reported that walking was helpful in preventing and easing symptoms of depression. Depression is a common disorder seen by physicians and is twice as common in women than in men. The symptoms of depression (fatigue, lack of energy, sleeplessness, decreased appetite, decreased sexual interest, weight change, constipation, lethargy, feelings of hopelessness, inability to function at home and at work, and mood changes among other symptoms), often bring many people to their primary care physician. Depressed individuals are also more likely to develop cardiovascular disease then non-depressed people.

Many recent studies have documented the benefits of exercise on mood in both healthy and clinically depressed individuals. Most of these studies have found exercise to have psychological and physiologic benefits for depressed people. In two separate studies using walking or strength-training exercises, participants in both groups were less depressed than the control group at the end of the trial and at later follow-ups. Exercise benefits have also been seen in people who are not clinically depressed but are at high risk for depression, for example college students who had a high number of stressful life events, female executives who are under considerable pressure at work and women who have considerable stress at home, especially those attempting to juggle work along with home responsibilities.

Psychologically, exercise may enhance one's sense of mastery, which is important for both healthy and depressed women who feel a loss of control over their lives. Exercise contributes to an improvement in self-esteem and may provide a therapeutic distraction from areas of worry, concern and guilt. In addition, improving one's health, physique, fitness, and weight may all enhance mood. Another benefit is that large-muscle activity may help discharge feelings of pent-up frustration, anger and hostility.

There are also mood-regulating effects of exercise on the neurochemistry of the brain. Exercise, particularly walking, may exert its beneficial effects on mood, by influencing the metabolism and increasing the availability of certain neuro-transmitters in the brain, in particular brain serotonin. An increase in brain serotonin exerts an antidepressant effect similar to the effects of antidepressant medications. Several other studies on brain chemistry have linked the ability of exercise to increase brain chemicals (beta-endorphins), which have a mood-elevating effect and can help to abate the symptoms of depression. Other studies have linked an elevation of *corticotropin-releasing hormone* (CRH) following exercise which also has a mood-enhancing effect.

It should be noted that people with symptoms of depression should be evaluated and treated by their own personal physician. The physician, if she/he thinks it's necessary may in turn refer the patient to a mental health care specialist for further evaluation and treatment. Depression can be a serious condition if not treated properly and in a timely manner. The primary treatments for depression, however, should not present any obstacles to exercising. Walking is an excellent choice for depressed patients because its mood-enhancing effects are proven, it is easily accessible, and it can be done with partners, making it a more pleasurable experience. (The Physician and Sports Medicine Oct. 1998, vol. 25, No. 10: 55-61.)

IT'S SMART TO WALK!

Women who walk regularly are less likely to experience memory loss and other brain function declines that can be associated with aging. These findings were presented at a meeting of the American Academy of Neurology on May 9, 2001. This research entailed the study of approximately 6000 women ages 65 and older. All of these women were given cognitive function testing at the beginning of the study and again after eight years. Women who walked the most demonstrated less memory loss than those in the lower exercise groups, even after adjusting for age and other coexisting medical conditions.

Researchers feel that there is a significant correlation between physical activity and chemical activity in the brain. As we saw in the previous study on depression, exercise has the ability to increase the availability of certain brain neuro-transmitters (serotonin) and mood-elevating brain chemicals (beta-endorphins). There can be little doubt, then, that women who walk regularly have better brain function as they age.

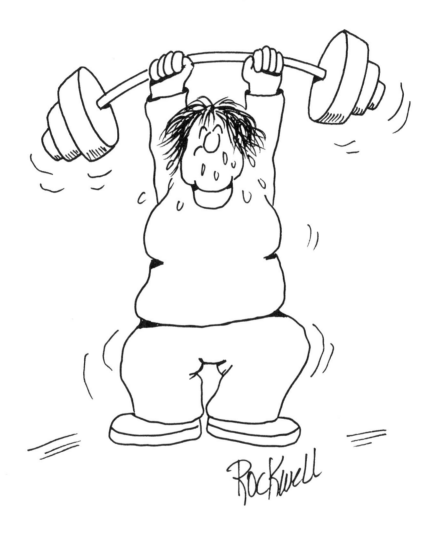

CHAPTER 12

TRIM-STEP®: FIT, FIRM, FABULOUS YOU!
****
A FIGURE SUPREME & A BODY THAT'S LEAN

Strength training is essential for weight control, muscle strengthening, skeletal health and overall well being in women. Aerobic exercise is great for cardiovascular health and burning calories, but it does not necessarily build upper body muscle strength. Fat replaces muscles as women age, unless they exercise to offset this natural process. The necessity for strength training is even more pronounced in women because they begin with more fat cells and less muscle tissue compared with men.

Women after the age of 35 lose muscle mass at a rate of approximately $1/3$ to $1/2$ pound per year. Strength training exercises, using light weight, hand-held weights while walking makes muscle stronger and strengthens the skeleton. The bones strengthen because the weights cause the muscles to contract. These muscle and ligaments then create a traction or tension on the bone, thus causing the bone to strengthen by absorbing more calcium from the blood-stream and losing less calcium from the bone. This process increases the mineral content of the bones, thus strengthening the bones and making them less brittle as you age.

Many studies have shown that women who engage in strength training exercises develop an increased skeletal muscle mass of approximately 1.5 kilograms, whereas sedentary women lose 0.5 kilogram muscle mass over a one year period. Likewise, bone mineral density increased by 1% in the strength training group and decreased by 2.5% in the sedentary group. Also, these studies showed that strength training women increased their lean muscle mass by 4% and decreased their fat mass by 8%.

What do all these numbers mean? They mean that your muscles will become more defined and shapely and you will feel stronger because your muscles are actually stronger. You will have better balance and greater joint flexibility. You will feel more energetic and more confident. Your bones will be structurally stronger and less likely to break as you get older. You will be less likely to develop osteoporosis or thinning of the bones as you get older. In other words, you will have *"a body that's lean and a figure supreme."*

TRIM-STEP®: STRENGTH TRAINING

Weight resistance exercises are not only good for your muscles but are also good for the body's most important muscle - the heart. In a recent report released by the American Heart Association, there is now increasing evidence that strength training can favorably modify many risk factors for heart disease, including blood cholesterol and triglycerides, blood pressure, body fat levels and glucose metabolism. Until recently, the conventional thinking was that strength training exercises helped to build and sculpt your muscles, but did little to help the cardiovascular system and in fact, might even be harmful to your heart. This current study released by the American Heart Association dispels many of the myths and misconceptions regarding strength training. The current study showed that strength training is not in the least harmful if one is reasonable and not trying to be a power weight lifter.

In addition to this special report by the American Heart Association which was published in the Journal of Circulation in February 2000, another related study was also released in February 2000 in the Journal of Hypertension. This study showed that weight strength training exercises can significantly lower blood pressure. Those women who regularly lifted light weights experienced a reduction in resting systolic blood pressure (when your heart muscles contract) and a reduction in the resting diastolic blood pressure (when your heart muscles relax). Their resting blood pressures dropped regardless of their body composition and whether they performed heavy weight resistance exercises with longer rest periods or lighter weight exercises with shorter rest periods. In other words using lighter weights as we suggest in the <u>Trim-Step® Walking Workout Plan</u> causes the same reduction in blood pressure as those people who are lifting heavier weights. Weight resistance exercises particularly using lighter weights as in the Trim-Step® Plan is safe and effective, unless, for example, you've had a previous heart attack, angina, high blood pressure, irregular heart rhythm or heart valve problems. In any event, everyone should have a complete physical examination before using hand-held light weights in the Trim-Step® Plan.

So you will see that the Trim-Step® Walking Workout Plan not only makes you feel and look great, but helps to strengthen your heart and lower your blood pressure. In addition, it sculpts and molds your body into a figure supreme and a body that's lean. Not a bad combination for a 20 minute walking workout twice a week.

TRIM-STEP® STEPS

1. <u>Work Out While You Walk.</u>

No matter how hard or long you walk, your upper body, particularly your arms, get a free ride. Upper body strength is only a small part of the walking motion. Even if you pump your arms vigorously the essential problem remains, which is that your arms don't get stronger since there is no resistance to encounter while you walk. This is unlike your legs in the Fit-Step program, which encounters the resistance of the ground and supports your body's weight. In other words your legs get stronger, your thighs, buttocks and hips get firmer and your abdomen gets flatter on the Fit-Step® plan.

Weight resistance with hand-held weights while walking is a great way to put your arms to work and at the same time makes you a stronger walker. A walker's upper body should be geared towards strength and endurance, not building muscle bulk. In other words we want to sculpt and mold the upper body (arms, back and chest). The key to the Trim-Step walking work-out plan is using light hand-held weights while walking, which provides strength training.

2. How Can Strength Training Exercises Help You Lose Weight?

When you walk with light hand-held weights you build muscle mass, which in turn speeds up your metabolism. Muscle tissue burns more calories than fat cells burn. Therefore building muscle helps to boost your resting metabolism. This increase in the resting metabolism occurs because of the actual increased muscle mass that you develop and the increased metabolic activity in the muscles themselves. When combining your twenty minute aerobic walk (Fit-Step®) with strength training exercises (Trim-Step®) you have the advantage of a "double blast" of calorie burning or weight loss while trimming and toning your body. First of all, the aerobic walking in the Fit-Step® plan burns approximately 360 calories per hour or 120 calories every twenty minutes. The strength training exercises in the Trim-Step® plan burn another 360 calories per hour or 120 calories every twenty minutes, which is accomplished just by increasing the body's basal metabolism. So you see you can actually lose more weight more quickly by walking with hand-held weights.

3. Won't Weight Training Make My Muscles Bulky Like A Man's?

Women are afraid to train like men for fear of developing

massive muscles. In reality, women don't have to fear turning into Arnold Schwartzeneger because of the increase in basal metabolic rate which occurs during the Trim-Step® strength training exercises. Remember this is not power weight lifting, this is a walking workout with hand-held weights.

Since women have more body fat than men, they are less likely to bulk up like men who have more muscle mass to begin with. Women will see improvement in muscle tone and strength after only four to six weeks on the Trim-Step® strength training exercises. Muscles will become more defined and sculptured for a trim, firm look.

4. How Often Should You Walk With Weights?

Studies show that strength training exercises 2-3 times per week prevents damage to muscle fibers that need time to regenerate (heal) after being stressed with weight resistance exercises. Also, varying the muscle groups during strength training exercises helps to provide strength benefits to all of the upper body's muscles on a graduated basis. The beauty of the Trim-Step® Strength Training exercises is that they are done while you are walking using very light weights. This decreases the possibility of muscle and ligament injury and eliminates the need for time-consuming regimented weight lifting routines. Newer research in exercise physiology has shown that working out a particular muscle group only twice a week offers the same strength and muscle toning benefits as working these muscles three times per week. What does this all mean? Well, on your Diet-Step® plan, which includes the Fit-Step® plan you will be walking six days per week. It will only be necessary to use hand-held weights on two days each week on your walking workout (Trim-Step®). If you desire more muscle toning and upper body strengthening exercises you can increase the walking workout with hand-held weights to three times per week.

5. How Many Repetitions Should You Do With Each Exercise?

As you'll see from the following six Trim-Step® Walking Workout Exercises, it is only necessary to use hand-held weights 2 days per week. You'll be able to customize the number of repetitions for each exercise depending on your own comfort level. Doing one set of 10-12 repetitions for each exercise is usually adequate as you rotate from one exercise to another. You can do more if your muscles don't become sore or if you don't tire easily. Remember to start slowly with fewer repetitions when you start your walking workout and gradually build up the number of repetitions until you reach your own comfort level. The American Heart Association's finding in their latest study showed that weight resistance exercises should be of moderate intensity. In other words instead of the fallacy "no pain-no gain," the truth as I've always stated is "train, don't strain."

The Trim-Step® Walking Workout Plan makes your body leaner and your muscles more defined and sculptured. In addition, this plan builds stronger bones and muscles, straightens your posture, and strengthens your joints and ligaments. The Trim-Step® Plan also boosts your metabolism which in turn helps you to lose weight. And finally strength training Trim-Step® exercises enhance your sense of well being and your self confidence. In other words, a new vital improved you will be full of pep when you do the Trim-Step®.

TRIM-STEP® WALKING WORKOUT EXERCISES

1. Natural Arm Swing Trim-Step®

This is the most common arm motion that you use when walking. Your arms hang down naturally at your side, holding weights with palms facing your body. As you walk, alternately swing your arms gently, as you bend your elbows slightly. This is the natural arm motion of walking that you use during your regular 6 day per week Fit-Step® walking plan. This exercise strengthens your triceps and upper shoulder muscles.

2. <u>Locomotive Arm Motion Trim-Step®</u>

This is the arm motion that you see joggers use while they are running. Hold your arms bent at approximately 90 degrees at the elbow. Hold weights with palms facing your body. Now, do the locomotive! Alternately move your arms forward and backward. You will feel the muscles of your upper arm, triceps and shoulder muscles strengthen as you do the locomotive.

3. <u>Hammer Curl Trim-Step®</u>

This exercise starts out like exercise number one (natural arm swing). Arms at your sides, holding weights with palms facing body. As you walk, bend each arm alternately at the elbow toward your shoulder, and then lower arm to the side of your leg. Pretend you're hammering a nail into a tabletop. This exercise strengthens your forearm and biceps muscles.

This exercise is safer to do while walking than is the traditional biceps curl, where your palms face away from your body. You prevent the hand-held weights from bumping your legs as you walk when you do the hammer curl instead of the traditional biceps curl. Also, you get better muscle strengthening and toning with this exercise.

4. <u>Flap Your Wings Trim-Step®</u>

Hold weights next to the sides of your legs, palms facing in. Lift both arms together, out to your sides and away from your body. Lift arms out to the level of your shoulders (no higher) as you walk, and then lower both arms to your sides. This exercise must be done carefully while you're walking, otherwise you may lose your balance or knock someone's head off that is abreast of you while you walk. If you find that this exercise is too difficult to do while walking, then wait until your walk is finished and then do 10-12 repetitions of the Flap Your Wings Trim-Step®. This exercise strengthens your upper back, chest and shoulder muscles.

5. Reach For The Sky Trim-Step®

Think of this exercise as lifting the world off your shoulders as you reach for the sky. Hold arms out to sides, elbows bent in line with chest. Hold weights in hands, palms facing forward at shoulder level. Now, reach for the sky! Raise weights above head, until arms are fully extended. Then lower weights back down to shoulder level. This exercise sculpts and strengthens the upper back and shoulder muscles.

6. Butterfly Trim-Step®

Hold weights in each hand in front of you at chest level, palms facing each other and elbows bent at 90 degrees. Raise both arms out to your sides like a butterfly. Then bring weights back together in front of you at chest level. Be careful not to bang your hands together. This exercise is particularly good for developing and sculpting mid chest and upper back muscles.

If you find this exercise is too difficult to do while walking, then you can do it at the end of your 20 minute walk. If you're tired, you can even do this exercise lying down as follows:

a. Lying on your back, with knees bent and feet on the floor.
b. Start with arms stretched out above you towards the ceiling with weights in each hand, with palms facing each other.
c. Slowly lower your arms out to the sides, and then pull arms back to starting positions. Use primarily your chest muscles

while doing this exercise, not your arm muscles.

TRIM-STEP® WORKOUT EXERCISE TIPS

1. Start with 1 pound weights for the first 4-6 weeks, and then build up to 2 pound weights after you are conditioned. If you find that 2 pound weights are too heavy, then stick with the 1 pound weights. You'll still get great muscle strengthening, toning and sculpting.

2. Tighten your abdominal muscles while you're doing these exercises. This helps to provide support for your upper body while toning and flattening your abdominal muscles.

3. You can vary the exercises as you walk. Remember to stop any particular Trim-Step® exercise if you become tired or your muscles become sore.

4. If you find that any of the exercises are too difficult to do while you walk (particularly exercises 4,5 and 6) then do them at the end of your walk. Only do 10-12 repetitions of each exercise while you are standing still.

5. The six Walking Workout Trim-Step® Exercises only have to be done 2 days per week to achieve maximum strength-training and muscle toning benefits. If the weather is bad, then these exercises can be done at home. Only do 10-12 repetitions of each exercise after your 20 minute indoor workout.

6. And lastly, how would you like to lighten your load (hand-held weights) as you continue on your 20 minute walk? Instead of hand-held weights, carry one 20-25 ounce plastic bottled water in each hand. As you proceed on your 20 minute walk, you can drink from each bottle alternately, until each bottle becomes lighter and lighter. When you're finished with your workout, you will be refreshed and rehydrated.

TRIM-STEP®: BEACH TONING

It is possible to almost double the number of calories that you burn when you are walking on sand rather than on hard surfaces. The reason for this is that your feet sink below the surface of the sand and your muscles, ligaments and joints have to work harder to lift your feet out of the sand. During your twenty minute walk it is possible to burn an additional 100-150 calories by just walking on sand.

Muscle toning in the areas of the calves, thighs, buttocks, and abdomen is more efficient on sand than just walking on hard surfaces. Again the reason for this is that the walking workout is more intense. Sand walking is great for beach toning which will enable you to look great in your bathing suit.

Wear a low cut walking sneaker to protect your feet from shells, rocks, glass and other beach debris. Keep your feet dry with light weight socks to protect against blisters; however, if you are brave enough, then walking barefoot can be a lot of fun if you are careful. Don't forget to use a good sun blocker to protect your skin from the sun's ultra-violet rays. Also be careful if you have any back, knee or ankle problems because of the excess strain put on these areas by the force transmitted by sand walking, which is a high intensity type of walking. Also the uneven walking surfaces that you encounter on sand sometimes can have an adverse effect on these problem areas. Stop if you develop pain in any area of the body and begin again after you've rested. You may tire more easily because of the increased difficulty of walking in sand. If that is the case, stop and rest and then begin again.

FIT-STEP®/ TRIM-STEP® BODY SHAPING PLAN.

Women are structurally built for walking, but not for running. Since the runner pounds the ground with a force equal to three to four times her body weight, she is more likely to sustain injuries than the walker. Walking is one of the most natural functions of the human body. Due to the structure of a woman's musculo-skeletal system and the shape and flexibility of her spine, her body is perfectly constructed for walking.

As you walk, the muscular and skeletal systems perform synchronously together. Your curved flexible spine has a spring-like function, made up of many vertebrae, each separated from the other by a tiny cushion (intervertebral disc), which is designed to absorb shock. These discs also give the spine its resilience and flexibility. When you walk, you use the hinge-like joints in your feet, ankles and knees while the ball and socket joints in your hips move effortlessly with a liquid-like motion.

The muscles that are attached to the long bones of the legs and the pelvis are specifically designed for walking. The leg, hip and back muscles are used for support and the mechanics of propelling the body forward. The long bones of the legs form a framework of levers which are moved by these muscles, and subsequently help to propel the body forward. The abdominal muscles support the weight of the abdominal organs when you walk and your chest wall and diaphragm muscles assist in respiration.

As your legs thrust forward, you are in effect catching the forward motion of the upper part of your body. This natural motion in walking creates a perfect balance between gravity's force and the forward thrust of your body. The act of walking is therefore an almost effortless bio-dynamic mechanism, structurally more efficient than any woman-made machine. Just remember to swing your arms naturally when you walk. If you want to exaggerate the swing more forcefully to burn more calories, and to shape your upper body, then use your hand-held weights. By combining your Fit-Step® walking plan with your Trim-Step® workout plan you have the perfect body-shaping plan.

BE A LEAN, MEAN, WALKING MACHINE

Walking produces a remarkable number of changes that occur inside of your body. Your *blood volume* and the red blood cells increase in number. Your *heart* pumps blood more efficiently. Your lungs expand, taking in and distributing more oxygen. Your muscles *tighten* and contract giving you a *firmer figure.* Your energy level increases, and you feel strong and fit. The results of these changes will make your *figure lean* and your *posture supreme.*

Your overall appearance will improve following your daily walk, since walking will improve your circulation and enable you to feel and look great. Your skin, complexion and hair texture will also improve with walking because of the increased blood circulation to the skin and hair follicles. Your complexion will literally glow after your walk and your skin will stay healthy and fresh looking all day long.

After you have been walking for awhile you will notice that your *muscles will become* firm and many of the fatty deposits on your thighs and buttocks will start to decrease in size. Your stomach will become flatter and the muscles of your *calves, thighs and buttocks* will become firmer and more shapely. These changes result from improved muscle tone and also from the strengthening of muscles and ligaments which are attached to the spine.

You don't have to kill yourself to stay fit, trim and healthy. Walking actually provides better long-term figure control and fitness benefits than jogging or other strenuous exercises, without the hazards and dangers. Always remember that exercise does not have to be painful or uncomfortable to be effective. The Fit-Step®/Trim-Step® Body Shaping plan provides the easy steps needed for a trim, beautiful body. *Be lean! Be mean! Be a walking machine!*

WALKING WOMEN UNITE!

Osteoporosis is a serious debilitating disease affecting over 20 million Americans, mostly women over the age of 45. This condition is actually a degeneration of bone throughout the body resulting in a loss of bone density. The bones actually become thinned-out as a result of a loss of the mineral calcium from the bone structure. Osteoporosis is especially marked after menopause because of a reduction in the secretion of estrogen by the aging ovaries.

Osteoporosis leads to approximately 1½ million fractures each year. Fractures of the hips are particularly common in older women. Approximately one out of five older women who sustains a hip fracture dies of secondary complications. This results in almost 35,000 deaths every year, making osteoporosis a leading cause of death among senior citizens. Another 25% of these women who break their hips become permanently crippled. Other serious complications of osteoporosis are fractures of the spinal column. These fractures can cause a collapse of the spinal vertebrae resulting in a shortening of actual height, a severe curvature of the spine ("dowager's hump"), or a paralysis of the spinal cord.

There are many therapies that are currently undergoing investigation for the treatment of osteoporosis. The most common form of treatment is the use of calcium supplements and hormonal replacement therapy. These and other recommended treatments have to be tailored to each woman, by her own physician. What do you think are the most important ways to prevent osteoporosis? *Walking and weight-bearing exercises lead to stronger bones and less chance of fractures.*

In a recent study reported in The *Journal of Orthopedic Research,* women who remained physically active after menopause or after age 50 had stronger, denser bones. Compared with inactive women ages 50-75, the active women had considerably greater arm and spine bone density measurements, almost in the same range as women 10-15 years younger. This study supports earlier research that shows that *osteoporosis* (thinning of the bones) can be slowed or halted by a regular walking program combined with weight-resistance exercises and that the incidence of bone fractures is 10 times less frequent in walking women. The Fit-Step®/ Trim-Step® Plan not only makes your muscles grow, but it also stimulates the growth of the bones under the muscles.

Walking outdoors when the sun is shining also helps to strengthen bones, because sunshine helps the body produce vitamin D, a nutrient needed for calcium absorption. And if these walking women ever do have the misfortune to break a bone - *their bones unite (heal) faster!*

DROP IN, NOT OUT!

Why are there so many exercise dropouts? And why don't many women even try to begin an exercise plan in the first place? Most women in these categories think that an exercise program is futile, since they'll never be able to look like the perfect bodies in the magazines or at the gym. They actually give up before they even start exercising, because of being intimidated.

Most women think physical fitness is actually harder than it is. And they feel that exercise programs are too complicated, when they hear terms like "oxygen consumption," "body fat composition," "body mass index," "lean muscle mass," etc. It all sounds too complicated and too boring for most women to begin exercising in any formalized program.

What most women don't realize is that you don't have to participate in a regimented exercise program to see results. They don't have to join a gym or health club and be intimidated by a twenty-year-old fitness instructor with boundless energy. And they don't have to exercise vigorously or do strenuous exercises in order to obtain maximum fitness and a lean, trim body. As we've already discussed, exercise doesn't have to be strenuous to see results. Exercise doesn't have to be painful in order to be gainful. You don't have to be put into a situation where you feel intimidated by an instructor in a gym or on a videotape.

Exercise can really be fun! It can be easy to follow and easy to continue. It doesn't have to be boring or a drudgery that has to be done. That's why the Fit-Step®/ Trim-Step® plan was devised - in order to make it easy for women to become fit and trim, and to make it easy for them to maintain their new level of fitness. Remember the two exercise myths we've discussed in the previous chapters - ("No Pain - No Gain" and the "Target Heart Rate Zone"). Both of these so-called exercise precepts are what makes many women discontinue their exercise plans or never start them in the first place. Once you realize that both of these so-called precepts are myths and that it is not necessary to make exercise painful or stressful, you can begin to begin to relax and enjoy the <u>Fit-Step®/ Trim-Step® Body Shaping Plan</u>.

WHAT'S THE BEST TIME TO DO THE FIT-STEP®/ TRIM-STEP® ?

You can do your walking aerobic workout exercise any time of the day that's convenient for you. It's your schedule, so make it any time that you'd like. You can also change the times that you exercise each day depending on your own individual work schedule or home activities. Here are the pros and cons of exercising at various times of the day according to the so-called fitness experts. Take it with a grain of salt and individualize your own schedule to your own liking.

<u>Morning</u> - The main obstacle in the morning is getting out of bed. Once you're up, depending on if you're an early riser or not, you may want to leave yourself enough time so that you won't be rushed, especially if you have to go to work or have home responsibilities. Since there are usually few disruptions in the A.M., women who walk in the morning are more likely to stick with their exercise plans over a long period of time. Plus, the sense of accomplishment, having completed your exercise early in the day, gives you a psychological rush for the first part of the day.

<u>Afternoon</u> - Many people feel an energy lag between two and three P.M. in the afternoon, which is related to the body's natural circadian rhythm. It may also be partly due to having just eaten lunch. Some exercise physiologists say that walking mid-day can smooth out that energy lag by increasing the levels of certain hormones that will perk you up for several hours. Remember, however, that it is not a good idea to exercise immediately after lunch or to skip lunch altogether. Walking for 20 minutes and then eating a light lunch will boost your energy level for the rest of the day.

<u>Evening</u> - Due to fluctuations in biological rhythms, it is in the late afternoon or early evening when your breathing is easier because your lungs' airways open wider, your muscle strength increases due to a slightly higher body temperature, and your joints and muscles are at their most flexible. This may also be a good time to walk according to some exercise physiologists. However, if you've had an extremely difficult day, and if you're dead tired, then revving yourself up for exercise may seem more like a chore than fun. Also, never exercise near bedtime, since the increased energy levels that follow the exercise may make it difficult to fall asleep.

Remember, however, that the choice is yours. Do the Fit-Step®/

Trim-Step® according to your own biological clock and how you feel, and also according to your own time schedule. It's your body, so listen to it, and it will respond to you with boundless energy and pep when you do the Fit-Step®/ Trim-Step®.

IT TAKES LONGER TO GET OUT OF SHAPE THAN IT DOES TO GET IN SHAPE

What if I can't keep up with the exercise plan regularly? What if I have to stop for a few days or a week or even longer if some interruption in my life prevents me from continuing? This is the kind of thinking that prevents many women from starting an exercise program and prevents others from going back to one that they've already begun. Never fear, the answer's here - *"It takes much longer to get out of shape than it does to get in to shape."*

The Fit-Step®/ Trim-Step® plan is forgiving. Even if you miss a few days or a week or a few weeks in a month, there is no need to worry. Once you have been conditioned physically, it takes a lot longer to get out of shape than it took you to get into shape. The rate of regression depends on how long you've been exercising and how fit you are. The body is remarkable, since it tends to hold on to these fitness gains long after you've stopped exercising. Most women lose muscle strength at about at about $1/2$ the rate at which they gained it. So, if you've been doing the The Fit-Step®/ Trim-Step® plan for three months, and have to discontinue for any reason, it could take up to six months for your body to fall back to its pre-training state.

Aerobic capacity starts to decrease in the first two to three weeks after you've stopped exercising, but it can take almost six to eight months before fit exercisers get back to the fitness level where they started. Aerobic exercising (walking) decreases the LDL (bad cholesterol) and increases the HDL (good cholesterol) after you've been on your walking program for approximately two to three weeks after you've stopped exercising, but it can take almost six to eight months befcre fit exercisers get back to the fitness level where they started. Aerobic exercising (walking) decreases the LDL (bad cholesterol) and increases the HDL (good cholesterol) after you've been on your walking program for approximately two to three months. Studies show that it took at least three months for these cholesterol levels to return to their original pre-walking workout levels after the exercise of walking was discontinued. That's pretty good, considering you've stopped walking all that time. When walkers resume their walking program, it took them only one-half the time to return to their original levels of fitness.

So, don't worry if you have to discontinue your walking pro-gram for any reason or for any period of time. The benefits that you've worked so hard for are long lasting and they are easily obtained again in one half the time. The Fit-Step® / Trim-Step® plan is forgiving and it keeps on giving!

TRIM-STEP®: STRETCH STEP

Stretching exercises can improve the flexibility of the joints, muscles and tendons, thus making the body less prone to injury. Stretching also increases the flow of blood to the stretched muscle and helps to promote bone growth where there is a stretching motion against gravity. There is increasing evidence that stretching has a calming effect on the central nervous system by transmitting relaxing signals along chemical neuro-transmitter pathways from the peripheral nervous system to the brain.

Stretching should be done slowly, and stretching one muscle group at a time is preferable. For instance, stretch both arms in front of you, and hold that position for 30 seconds and then let your arms down slowly, and relax them for an additional 30 seconds. Repeat this extension of both arms out to your sides, holding for 30 sec-onds, and then slowly letting them down and relaxing them for 30 seconds. Repeat this motion with your arms above your head, and then with your hands clasped in back of your head with your elbows bent, as if you are stretching when you get out of bed.

During each of these exercises, gently stretch the arms, by actually pulling or pushing them away from the body, and then pulling them back towards the body. Remember to do it gently, and if it hurts, you're stretching your muscles too much.

Do the same procedure with your neck muscles. First look up and hold your head in that position for 30 seconds and then relax, returning to a normal head position for 30 seconds. Repeat the same procedure looking to the left, and then to the right. Also, repeat this looking down, with your chin resting on your chest for 30 seconds, and then return to the normal head position for 30 seconds.

The best way to stretch your leg muscles and ligaments is to sit in a chair and stretch one leg at a time in front of you for 30 seconds, then relax the muscles, and then bend your knee, and hold that position for an additional 30 seconds, then relax the muscles and place your foot back on the floor. Repeat the same procedure with the other leg. You also can accomplish the same thing by pressing your feet into a foot-rest while sitting on a plane, train, bus, or at your desk.

These simple stretching exercises are designed to develop maximum flexibility of the muscles, ligaments and joints. Although not as elaborate as yoga or tai-chi, they are effective limbering and toning exercises for the body. These stretching steps help prepare the body for mental as well as physical fitness. These exercises help you to get in touch with your body as you contemplate the slow relaxing, stretching steps. Remember also to take slow deep breaths during the stretching exercises for maximum relaxing techniques.

You can develop any stretching routine that feels good to you, not just those described above. Stretching is an individual exercise, and what feels good for one person may not be satisfactory to another person. Stretching can be done also by interlacing the fingers in front of your body, above your head or behind your back.

Remember, if the stretching exercise hurts, either during or after the exercise, then you have stretched too vigorously. Go easy the next time. When you've finished, your muscles should feel relaxed, not taut or tight. The major advantage of the Stretch-Step is that it can be done any time, anywhere or any place. When you don't have the time to walk or the weather's inclement, stretching is a viable alternative to limbering up. Stretching can also be used in conjunction with the Fit-Step®/ Trim-Step®Plan.

TIGHT ABS/TRIM THIGHS/FIRM BUNS

Tell most people that walking produces a flat tummy, slim hips and thighs and they'll tell you that you're crazy. "You need to do strenuous calisthenics and exercises to reduce fat deposits in those areas." Don't be too sure! Walking can give you a flat, firm tummy and slim hips and thighs without any additional exercises. However, when you also do the Trim-Step® Walking Workout Exercises, you'll quickly develop a trimmer more sculptured figure.

First of all, when you walk briskly with an even stride you are contracting and relaxing muscles in your chest, back and abdomen. With each forward motion of your legs, these muscles contract to keep your body erect. Your abdominal muscles tighten automatically, exactly as they would if you were doing strenuous sit-ups, with one exception - you're not straining your back muscles. As you swing your upper arms, the upper chest wall muscles that are tied in with the upper abdominal wall muscles aid in tightening these abdominal muscles. This combination of upper body and lower abdominal muscle contractions is what produces a *firm, flat tummy*. With repeated bouts of walking come repeated bouts of muscle tightening, until a point is reached when your abdominal muscles are firm and taut all of the time, whether you're walking or not. This firm, flat tummy will continue to last as long as you walk regularly. Also as you walk, the forward and backward motion of each hip stretches the hip muscles. This hip motion tugs at your lower abdominal muscles, further fattening your tummy

Now what about those lumpy, bumpy hips and thighs. First of all, don't let anyone give you the baloney about *"cellulite deposits."* There's no such thing as cellulite! It's a term coined by diet promoters to encourage people to purchase diet-gimmicks to rid themselves of the mythical cellulose. Microscopic studies of fat show that fat cells are connected by strands of connective tissue. When these connective tissue strands stretch, they lose their elasticity and subsequently the fat gives a lumpy appearance. Regular fat cells and the so-called cellulite fat deposits are indistinguishable under the microscope. *Fat is fat!* And cellulite is phoney-baloney! Again, walking regularly combined with weight-resistance exercises will trim down those lumpy, bumpy hips and thighs.

Let's get back to developing *thin and trim thighs*. When you walk briskly your pelvis shifts forward and your buttock muscles contract as you stride forward. Your lead leg pulls you forward as your back leg pushes you forward. Both of these motions contract and relax your leg muscles both in front and in back of your thighs. This alternate flexing and relaxing of the thigh muscles tones and trims your thighs better than any machine can do and with considerably less likelihood of injury. Repeated regular bouts of brisk walking also burns away fat deposits in your thighs. Since walking is a moderate aerobic exercise, it burns fat rather than muscle tissue. The result: *trim and thin thighs*. When this walking fat-burning process is combined with weight-bearing exercises, you will also lose those unsightly bumpy and lumpy (the mythical cellulite) fat deposits. Sounds too easy? It certainly is! It's the Fit-Step®/ Trim-Step® Body Shaping Plan.

O.K. let's get on to those *wide-spread hips and flabby buttocks*. Now I know you'll say that you inherited those from your mother or your grandmother and there's nothing you can do about it. Well, I'll tell you that you didn't inherit those characteristics from anyone. First of all, your mother and your grandmother probably never did much walking at all, let alone any weight-bearing exercises, and that's why they had wide bottoms and fat hips. Too much sitting is bad for the derriere and the hips. Inactivity in these areas leads to the accumulation of fatty deposits and the loss of connective tissue elasticity. These factors combine to give what's known as the spread-hip, wide-bottom look. Not a look designed for today's modern womens' fashions. You don't have to accept it as inevitable. You don't have to contend with flabby buttocks and hips, even if you've already got them.

Walking and strength-training exercises will prevent flabby hips and thighs and a wide, droopy bottom. Don't let anyone tell you that they're permanent. As you walk briskly your upper legs and hips stretch forward and backwards with each stride that you take. Your hips and buttocks also move from side to side by rotating, as your legs swing forward. This motion tightens your hip and buttock muscles, which starts the slimming process almost immediately. The forward motion of your legs combined with the tightening of the lower abdominal muscles also produces a tightening effect of your lower back and buttocks muscles. This combination of alternate muscle groups contracting and relaxing produces firm, tight buttocks muscles. This firming effect actually lifts the buttocks so that they lose their saggy appearance. Your thighs will also become thin and trim and will remain that way as long as you continue the Fit-Step® / Trim-Step® Body Shaping Plan.

FIT, FIRM, FABULOUS YOU!

You will start to develop a sprightly step as you do the Fit-Step®/ Trim-Step®. Your stride will become smooth and effortless as you thrust your legs forward, and you will begin to feel a lively spring and bounce with every step that you take. This walking method helps to stimulate the circulation throughout the entire body. As you walk, your chest will expand, providing more room for your heart and lungs to work efficiently. Your stomach muscles will tighten, supporting your internal organs properly in the fashion that they were accustomed to being supported when your abdominal muscles were in their prime.

Your posture will improve as your shoulders find their way back to their upright position. Your head will assume the erect position and your back and spine will straighten like the shoot of a young branch. Your buttocks and thigh muscles will tighten and firm up, and your upper arms will lose their flabby appearance. Your figure will slowly go through a metamorphosis and you will appear younger, feel better and be healthier than you ever were before. You will actually slow down the aging process to the point at which you will look and feel 10-15 years younger. Your weight will decrease as you travel the Fit-Step®/ Trim-Step® plan. You will *burn steam as your energy beam keeps you lean with a figure supreme.*

Walk off weight, walk off worry, walk off stress and tension as you walk away the years and the ravages of aging. This program will give you a perfect body as you feel and look younger. I guarantee you a better figure, a leaner body and a fit, trimmer you. Don't give in to the ravages of the aging process. Don't let inactivity sap your bones of their calcium, your muscles of their strength and your body of its life. Don't let your body start to sag before its time. Use your only defense available against the aging process - walking every day the Fit-Step®/ Trim-Step® way.

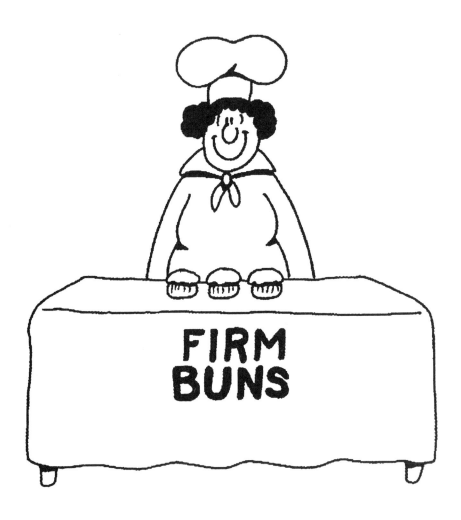

INDEX

****

MEDICAL MANOR BOOKS ® :QUICK ORDER FORM

Postal orders:
Medical Manor Books, 3501 Newberry Rd., Philadelphia PA 19154

Telehone orders :
Call:800-DIETING (343-8464) Toll Free.

Fax orders:
215-440-WALK (9255).

E-mail orders:
medicalmanor@aol.com

Web site orders:
www.medicalmanorbooks.com (or) www.diet-step.com

<All major credit cards accepted>

The following books by the author are available from Medical Manor Books ®

Title of Book		Price
Walk,Don't Run	ISBN: 0-934232-00-8	$ 6.95
DIETWALK® (Paper)	ISBN: 0-934232-02-4	$ 8.95
Walk,Don't Die (Cloth)	ISBN: 0-934232-06-7	$18.95
Walk,Don't Die (Paper)	ISBN: 0-934232-05-9	$ 9.95
Walk to Win (Cloth)	ISBN: 0-934232-08-3	$19.95
Walk to Win (Paper)	ISBN: 0-934232-07-5	$10.95
Dr. Walk's® Diet & Fitness Newsletter (Quarterly)		$24.95
DIET-STEP®:20/20 (Cloth)	ISBN: 0-934232-10-5	$25.95
DIET-STEP®:20/20 (Paper)	ISBN: 0-934232-09-1	$15.95

Shipping by air :

      US: $3.95 for 1st book and $1.95 each additional book

      International: $9.95 for 1st book and $ $4.95 each additional book

      Sales tax: Add 6% for books shipped to Pennsylvania addresses